201 Homemade Beauty Tips & Tricks

201 Homemade Beauty Tips & Tricks

Release
The Gypsy and the Belle
In You

Thato Gaboitsiwe

201 Homemade Beauty Tips and Tricks: Release the Gypsy and the Belle in You

Copyright © 2015 by Thato Gaboitsiwe

ISBN-13: 978-1499533033

ISBN-10: 1499533039

Please note that the effectiveness of each product differs from one person to another and that the benefits may be limited to one or two skin types thus a remedy may work for people with oily skin but not work for those with dry skin type. It is advisable to perform spot tests, especially if you are aware that you have sensitivity to particular products to avoid allergy reactions.

Disclaimer

201 Homemade Beauty Tips & Trips: Release the Gypsy and the Belle in You book is provided for general informational purposes only. The opinions expressed here are the author's and not those of any advertiser, company, affiliate or group.

None of the content or opinions are meant to harm or malign any religion, ethnic group, club, organization, company or individual.

The information contained in this book is for general information purposes only. The information is provided by the author and while the author made an effort to keep the information up to date and correct, the author makes no representations or warranties of any kind, express or implied, about the completeness, accuracy, reliability, suitability or availability with respect to the book or the information, products, services or related graphics contained in the book for any purpose. Any reliance you place on such information is therefore strictly at your own risk. The book is provided "as is", without warranty of any kind, either express or implied, and your use of the book constitutes your consent to these terms.

This content is not intended to diagnose or treat any disease, or as a substitute for medical advice. Only a qualified health professional may diagnose disease, therefore self-treatment of symptoms of illness is not advisable. Please consult with your advising physician before for starting any treatment for a medical condition. The author, publishers, and distributors of this work shall not be held liable or responsible for any misunderstanding or misuse of the information contained on this site or for any loss, damage, or injury caused or alleged to be caused directly or indirectly by any treatment, action, or application of any herbs, products, food or food source discussed in this site. In no event will the author or the publisher, be liable for any consequential, incidental or direct damages suffered in the course of using the information in this book.

The information in this book is only for educating the reader. It is not meant to substitute the advice of a medical professional. If you are suffering from a serious health condition, please see a medical expert as soon as possible.

Images credit: pixabay.com

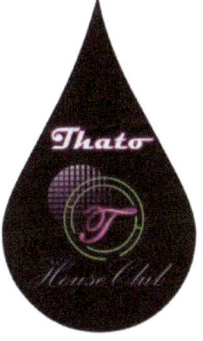

Dedications

To all the beautiful women and men around the world

Beauty is an opinion and optional. It's how you estimate yourself that defines your level of beauty.

Beautiful Woman

Oh woman how merry you make me
Drank in your beauty you leave me bowled over
Only you do not know how bewitching your looks are
Many are the princes drowning in your splendour

Grace you were born with
Charmed are all the fine men by your elegance
Maidens sing your praises
Come now pleasure yourself in your birth right

Let us dance the night through
To the song that is held by our hearts
I request only to divulge your alluring, slumbering looks
Your beauty is a windfall to all gentlemen

Thato Gaboitsiwe

Acknowledgement

To my precious gem: D'or Ame Mimi Mushure, with love.

I wish to acknowledge the invaluable assistance and guidance of a number of people in the course of completing this venture.

I appreciate the support of my closest and best friend, supporter and confidante, Edmore Mushure, for his unwavering belief in my ability – You found the beauty in me even when I doubted myself at times.

I owe an unquantifiable, intellectual debt to Zibo Molefe.

With the deepest gratitude I wish to acknowledge the following people:

Pulane Makhiwa – For motivating and believing in me.
Diphetogo Thomas – You've always made me realise the simplicity and beauty of laughter.
Tapiwa Morapedi – The beauty guru.
Pinkie Isabela – You really do inspire me.

For inspiring me and invaluable help: Stephen Mushure, Keitumetse Onana Faesone, Benjamin Khiriyone, Motshepi Kgomotso, Sethunya Ruda, Lechani Mabutho and Tebogo Dioka.

Finally, I am indebted to the artists, too numerous to mention, who unknowingly provided me with images that made this book attractive and easy to read.

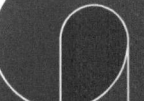

To

My Dearest Baby
My Little Bella

D'or Ame Mimi

Whenever you give me that innocent look and say, 'Mommy, you are beautiful.' And you pause and wait expectantly for the inevitable and yet much appreciated reply, 'Thank you my sunflower, you are beautiful too.' And you smile and say, 'Thank you.' It always brings about the butterflies in my stomach.

I hope that you never forget the two lessons from this simple, short yet empowering conversation:

1. Always believe in yourself, you might need assurance now and then from other people but know that no matter what, you're the biggest influence of your life.

2. See the good in other people, learn to appreciate others; if you're tempted to say a negative thing about another person, rather try and find one good thing about them and use that to either open or shut your mouth.

Love

xoxo

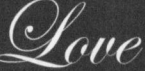

Table of Contents

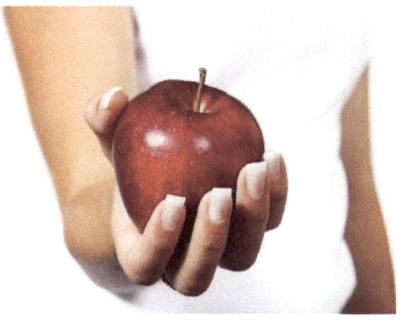

Foreword

A woman is crafted with so much care by the Master. She is a masterpiece that intelligent design doesn't even begins to describe her and her beauty. Being a woman is all about being a grandmother, wife, mother, aunt, sister and friend. Count the beautiful titles put on a woman and you would know she is *perfect*!

The beauty a woman carries within herself is hard to ignore as it shines through her, it is shown through many platforms, either in her community, society, at work, church, school and everything that she touches. Talking about the beauty of a woman cannot be all put just in one word or sentence, neither can we just conceal it nor can the biggest jar in the world contain it all, a more reason for a woman to shine. Different people have versions on what exactly is beauty, but mostly arrive to one answer; one word, 'woman'. And this here ladies, is a book specifically written for you to reclaim your title, you are the diamonds, and you know who you are; so it's time you utilise your confidence and carry yourselves that way. And so my dear diamonds, it's time to let our inner beauty shine on the outside too. There is nothing that beats confidence - confidence in self!!

Enjoy the home remedies and look fabulous, always.

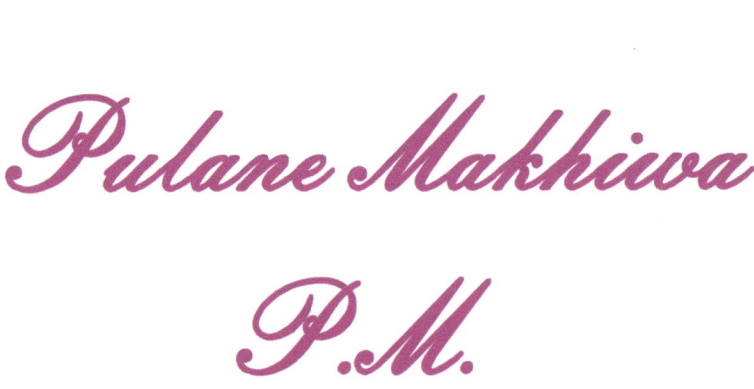

Pulane Makhiwa

P.M.

Preface

I passed through my teen years with a face under acne and zits torment. I never knew what to do with the war that was taking place on my face. My body had chosen to have a combination of oily skin on the face and dry skin in other parts. I tried different skincare products that promised miracles and most of them worked for a short period then afterward the inevitable war erupts. The only thing that really saved me back then was my high self-confidence or otherwise I would have locked myself up and never wanted to be seen with a battleground for a face.

My adulthood hasn't been anything different to what I had experienced when growing up. On top of things, I have always had a yoyo body weight. Tired of the no-food diet fads, one day I decided to lose weight in a healthy way and so started my research for healthy ways to do that. I was intrigued by one diet called GM diet (please note that the author does not have any affiliation with the owners of this diet being GM Motors). The diet recommends one to consume fruits and veggies all in their given day. I followed the diet religiously for 7 days and not only did I lose some weight in few days, I started to see my skin clearing up of the zits.

The fact that the diet consists of only natural food I started to wonder what more can mother nature offer me that will be also be appreciated by my body and my research started. I started to scratch my head for those old and forgotten beauty tricks that the elderly women used to tell us when we were young. I would ask some of my friends to try the tricks on them to see if they work and viola – the worked and so they idea to share these inexpensive and old beauty regimes was born and now ladies and gentlemen, girls and boys I present to you…

201 Homemade Beauty Tips & Tricks: The Gypsy and La Bella in You

This page intentionally left blank

Introduction

From the ancient age, women from all walks of the globe have always dedicated time to always look their best – both physically and mentally. This dedication to beauty resulted in women devoting their time and energy to come up with beauty regimes created from natural ingredients such as vegetables and fruits.

As time went by and women started to take on another role of being co-breadwinners, they started to have less and less time for themselves in between their professional lives and home chores. This gave birth to the beauty industry which promised women magnificent looks just by using their products.

The beauty products came already prepared and all the women had to do was to open the bottles or tubes and apply onto their skin without having to first slave away or better yet, go under the knife and come out looking a decade younger than their true age. All of these proved to be enticing to be ignored by most women and as such, the tradition of making one's own beauty products was thrown away and women started to rely heavily on commercially, synthetic-chemically endorsed products which usually contain countless ingredients some of which are harmful to our skin.

The sudden increase of women's dependence on chemically-produced beauty products meant that their power to decide on what they put on their skin was no longer with them by with the manufacturers. The fact that women nowadays are going back and consulting the olden beauty treatments comes as no surprise due to certain facts:

1. The fact that one can find a product that she so desires to use on her skin but only to find out it contains ingredients such as *denatured alcohol* or *acetone* in - it must be disheartening for many women.
2. Or maybe the fact that the beauty industry charges exorbitant prices for their products should be enough to discourage one to continue shelving the ancient skincare and other beauty regimes that had proven to have worked away any longer.

It is high time women re-learn and observe what women of earlier generations knew: nobody and nobody knows your skin better than you know it and as such, women should take their time and cook up the concoctions that will give them the exquisite looks that they so desire. The reality is that most of these homemade regimes do not cost much and the fact that the time taken to produce is them is short should be motivation on itself.

Eyes, Eyelashes, Brows, Teeth and Lips

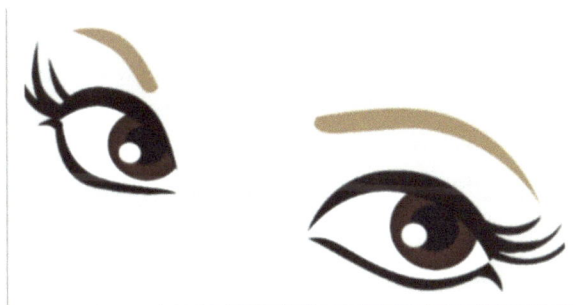

The eye is perhaps one of the most indispensable part of the human body. The eye feeds our brains with information regarding our surrounding and such, enabling the brain to make sound judgement regarding any situation. The eye is also a sensitive part so naturally extra care is needed to be provided at all times.

The eye is always exposed to harsh conditions which include ultraviolet radiation which accelerate eye conditions such as retinal damage, cataract and eye cancers.

Eyes, Eyelashes and Brows

The eyelashes and eyebrows are exposed to different external negative factors and treatments such as makeup cosmetics, makeup removers, dyes, threading, trimmed, waxed, plucked, shaved or sugared. Eyebrows prevent sweat, blood and other foreign liquid from the skin from getting into the eye and the eyelashes prevents dust and other particles from getting into the eyes.

Eyelashes and eyebrows are particularly used to boost people's physical looks more especially the healthy and thick ones. One of the basic rule of proper care of lashes and brows care is to press the cotton pads soaked in hair-friendly makeup removal for 10 seconds gently on them. For the eyelashes and eyebrows to perform their aesthetic and soothing functions, one needs to take proper care of them.

1. Use raw potato to cool and reduce puffy, baggy eyes. Peel the potato and cut it half then place them over your eyes for 10 minutes.

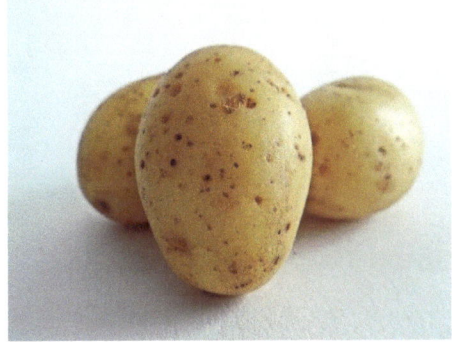

2. Get rid of puffy eyes with ice cubes of green tea. Make green tea, let it cool then pour it into ice maker, once the green tea has iced, take the an ice cube and massage under one eye until the ice cube melts then repeats on the other eye.

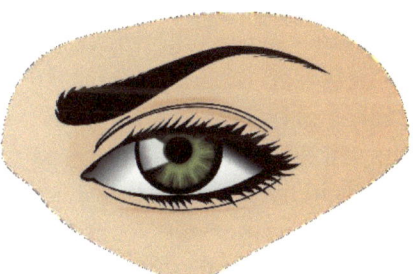

3. Cucumber juice can also be a solution to puffy eyes because of its high water content. Grate 1 cucumber then divide the fleshy tissues and juice equally, roll the contents up into 2 separate strips of gauze then put the strips onto the eyes. Another way to use cucumber is to slice it and place a slice on each eye for at least 10 minutes. Cucumber works well on eyes that have swelled or puffed due to hangover or after crying.

4. Dip a cotton ball in warm water and wipe your eyebrows before tweezing to soften the skin.

5. When tweezing your eyebrows, move the tweezers in the direction of where hair grows.

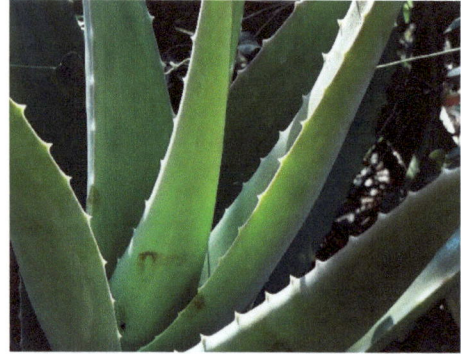

6. Use aloe vera gel or juice to de-puffy your eyes and improve blood circulation and as well as getting rid of excessive fluid around the eyes. Apply the gel or juice under your eyes and leave it on for the whole day.

7. Overindulgence of salty food is a no-no area but if you ever go down that road and have puffy eyes to show for it then salt can be a good friend. Put ½ teaspoon of salt into a glass of warm water then stir until the salt dissolves. Soak facial pads or cotton balls in the solution, squeeze out excess liquid and massage your eyes for about 2 minutes then lie down and place the cotton balls or pads on your eyes for about 10 minutes.

8. If your eyes have swollen or puffed due to lack of enough sleep, fill a small bag or plastic bag with ice and wrap it in a facecloth or frozen vegetable bag and place it over your eyes for 5-10 minutes. If you are out of ice, you can splash your face with cold water. The coldness helps to reduce swelling by constricting blood vessels. Repeat if necessary until the swelling disappears.

9. To avoid drawing a hard line on your eyebrows, do not use the pointed tip of a sharpened brow pencil rather use the side of the tip to make the line.

10. Use the tannic and gallic acids found in witch hazel to reduce eye inflammation. Soak cotton balls in witch hazel and place them on the eyes for 15-20 minutes.

11. The antibacterial and antiseptic properties found in rosewater help in cooling and lessening eye inflammation. Soak cotton balls in rosewater and place them on the eyes for 15-20 minutes.

12. To tame wild eyebrows, sprinkle hairspray to your old toothbrush and gently brush the eyebrows upward and outward.

13. For thicker, colour-rich and fast growing eyebrow hair, massage olive oil twice a day to your eyebrow hair. The Vitamin E found in olive oil nurtures the hair follicles.

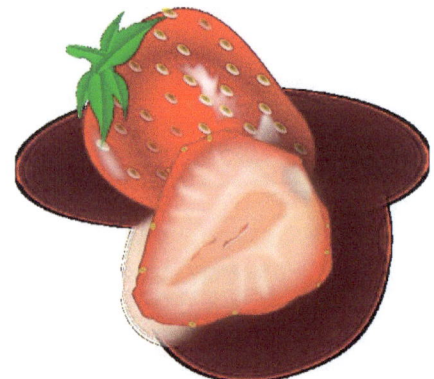

14. To reduce under-eye puffiness and swelling that comes with age, use strawberries. Strawberries contain alpha-hydroxy acids that assist to smoothen and tighten the skin under the eyes. Refrigerate strawberries for half an hour, cut off their tops then slice them into thick pieces. Put the slices under your eyes for at least 20 minutes.

15. To nourish and enhance eyebrow hair growth, apply castor oil to your eyebrows every night. Castor oil contains antioxidants, vitamins and protein which help in nurture eyebrow hairs.

16. Omega 3, Omega 6, Omega 9, lecithin and B vitamins can be found in flax seeds and therefore, its oil can assists in promoting eyelash growth and revamp them. Dab a drop of flax seed oil on your eyelashes every night before going to sleep.

17. Use aloe vera gel to de-puffy your eyes and improve blood circulation.

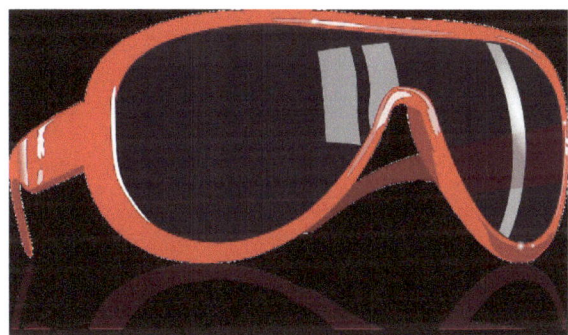

18. Always wear UV-blocking sunglasses if you are going to be exposed to the sun to protect your eyes from ultraviolet (UV) rays and also to reduce the sun's intense glare.

19. Massage pure aloe vera gel into your eyebrows to help them grow.

20. Apply haemorrhoid cream under your eyes to de-puffy your eyes. The anti-inflammatory agents found in the cream helps in relieving eye puffiness.

21. Use milk to soothe itchy eyes. Simply soak two cotton balls in cold milk and place them on your eyes to cool them or swap a cotton ball in cold milk and rub it around your eyes. Perform the remedy once in the morning when you wake up and in the evening before bed.

22. To get rid of dark circles around the eyes, use potatoes. Potatoes possess catechole enzyme which easily lightens the skin. Simply cut a potato into thin slices and store the slices in the fridge until they chill. Place the chilled slices onto your eyes for 10-15 minutes.

23. Crush fenugreek seeds and mix them with few drops of almond oil. Apply the mixture onto your eyebrows daily before bedtime and rinse off in the morning.

24. Use cotton bud to apply whole milk to your eyebrows on daily basis to assist them to grow thick.

25. Soak your facecloth in lukewarm rooibos tea and gently dab your eyes to treat sensitive, irritated and itchy eyes. Another way to treat itchy eyes is to place two wet rooibos tea bags over your eyes for 10-15 minutes.

Lips

26. Want smooth lips; put a drop of mustard oil in your belly button before bed. Weird but works.

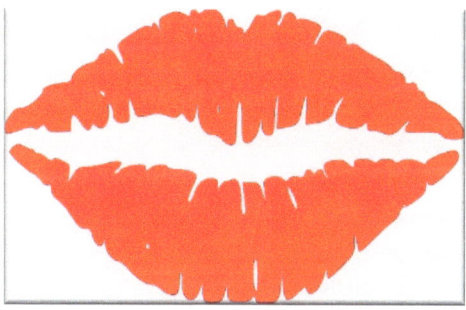

27. Use lemon juice as lip exfoliator. Gently rub the juice on your lips and leave it overnight then rinse it in the morning to get rid of dead skin cells. Do not use on broken or chapped lips.

28. Gently brush dry and cracked lips with your wet toothbrush to exfoliate and leave them silky and soft then apply your usual

lip balm. Avoid licking your lips at any given time.

29. For smooth and velvet lips, mix 2 teaspoons of coriander juice with 1 teaspoon of lemon juice. Rub in the ointment on your lips and leave it on overnight then wash if off in the morning. Repeat the treatment for several days for great results.

Teeth

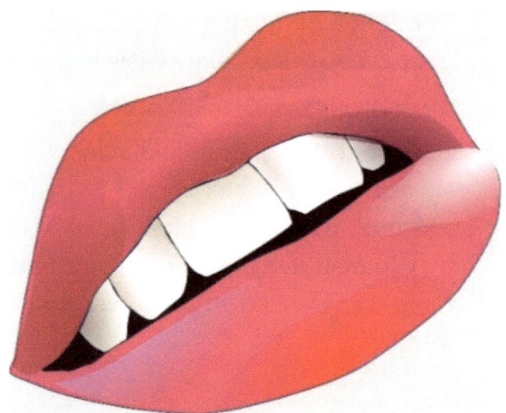

We use our teeth to chew food and they also helps us in forming words when we talk. Drugs and foods can cause teeth to discolour, decay, cavities, loose and crooked teeth and gum diseases. To prevent teeth diseases and to prolong a bright and white smile, one needs to take good care of their teeth and take oral health seriously by practising healthy habits such as properly brushing and flossing daily to reduce bacteria or plaque buildup and seeing their dentist every six months.

30. Lemon juice and baking soda can be used as natural teeth whiteners. Mix few drops of lemon juice with baking soda and apply the mixture to your teeth using cotton bud then scrub your teeth with toothbrush and rinse.

31. Mix 1 tablespoon of baking soda with 5 drops of hydrogen peroxide and a couple of water drops and mix well. Apply the solution to your teeth using your toothbrush and leave it for 5-10 minutes then brush your teeth with the toothbrush and rinse with water. Use the remedy once every week to whiten your teeth.

32. If it is not possible to brush your teeth after eating, try rinsing your mouth after eating to prevent food such as beetroots and other colourful foods from staining your teeth.

A good dental and eye care can help in the overall healthy condition of your body.

Face

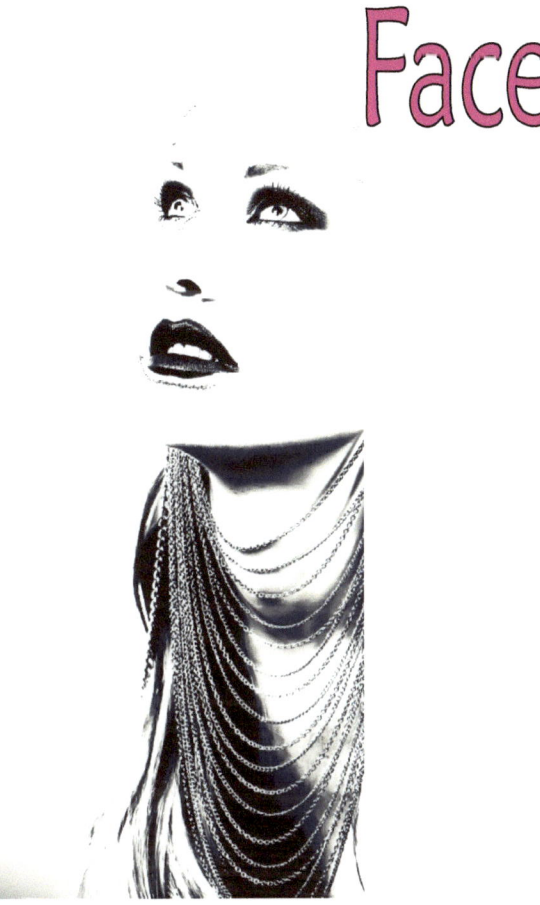

The human face has the ability to express emotions and moods. It is also one of the body parts that stand out the most and doubly is mostly remember part. The face has about thirty (30) facial muscles that participate to communicate our emotions. The facial muscles enable us to express our feelings without the need for words.

The face can also reveal the health status of a person as various diseases and health conditions are revealed in the face. It is of uttermost importance to take care of the face as it is exposed to harsh conditions most of the times. Our faces easily reveal our physical and mental health conditions.

33. To reduce the redness on your face from strenuous activities such as workouts, take an antihistamine.

34. Almond oil is rich in vitamins and minerals and as such makes a good makeup remover. Dap a little bit of oil on a cotton swab or wool and gently rub away the makeup such as foundations, cream, eyeliners, eye shadow or cream. It also exfoliates the skin at the same time.

35. The anti-inflammatory properties of grape seed oil assists in reducing the appearance of acne and also to heal pimples.

36. Pepto Bismol is used to break down acids and oil in the digestive system but did you know that it can work the same way on your face? The antibacterial active agent, bismuth subsalicylate, found in the anti-acid can be used to treat acne by tightening skin, dry out zits and shrink pores. Apply 2 tablespoons of Pepto Bismol on your face and leave it on for 20 minutes then raise it off with plain, warm water. Do not use it daily as it will dry out the skin.

37. Concealers are every girl's best friend when it comes to hiding flaws but sometimes too much can have the opposite effect of what one's trying to achieve. To get rid of zit immediately, use nasal spray or eye drops such as Clear Eyes, All Clear or Visine. These products contain vasoconstrictors which help in reducing blood vessels. Simply dab the affected area with spray or eye drops to reduce inflammation and eliminate redness.

38. Apply makeup then step into hot bath or near a hot shower for 10 minutes. The vapour assists in setting the makeup and leaving the skin looking renewed and striking gorgeous.

39. Use aloe vera gel or juice to keep zits at bay. Simply rub the gel from the aloe vera plant or pure aloe vera gel onto the pimples.

40. Rub one drop of lavender oil onto your zits and leave it on overnight then wash well in the morning.

41. Rub one drop of tea tree essential oil onto your zits and leave it on overnight then wash well in the morning. This helps to get rid of pimples.

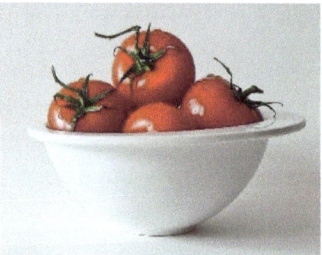

42. Squeeze a fresh tomato and massage the juice onto your face and leave it on onto your face for 1 hour then rinse it off.

43. Massage a slice of potatoes onto your zits and leave the juice on your skin for the whole day before washing it.

44. Use green tea as an astringent to alleviate the pimples. Pour green tea into ice maker and rub the ice cubes onto the affected area 3-4 times a day.

45. Mix castor oil with dried calendula e.g. marigold to relieve the inflammation.

46. Acne can be caused by hormonal imbalances in the body. Siberian Ginseng is known for its properties that assist in rebalancing hormonal abnormalities and boosting the immune system in our bodies. Taking Siberian Ginseng capsules helps in enhancing your skin and removing acne.

47. To unblock pores and scrub dead cells and make your skin smooth, pound a small amount of aspirin which contains salicylic acid known for unclogging pores and mix it with honey. Apply the mixture to your face and leave it for 30 minutes then rinse it off.

48. The astringent properties of witch hazel make it one of the remedy for blemish. Soak a cotton ball into witch hazel then place over the pimples.

49. Garlic has anti-inflammatory, antifungal, antibiotic, antimicrobial and antiviral properties and is also very rich in antioxidants which are helpful in getting rid of acne and free radicals and promotes resilient immune system. The antibacterial agent, allicin, found in the cloves has antifungal properties and assists in defending against harmful bacteria. Peel a clove of garlic and crush it to activate its composites. Massage the fleshy tissue to your zits and leave for 20 minutes before rinsing it off. You can also add the crushed garlic to your warm tea or eat it raw.

50. Place wet hibiscus onto your zits and hold it for at least 5 minutes.

51. Apply cucumber juice on your face to reduce the appearance of wrinkles.

52. Rub plain white toothpaste to a zit overnight to dry it out. Avoid toothpaste made from gel.

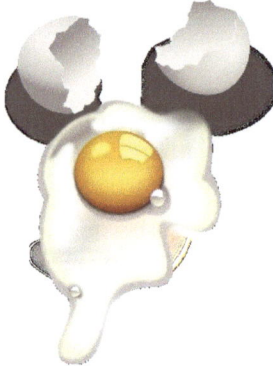

53. For glowing face skin, rub the egg white on to your face and leave overnight. In the morning wash well with warm water.

54. For bright and firm skin, pound a handful of pomegranate seeds with cherries then massage the puree into your face. Leave it for 10 minutes to allow their natural enzymes to enhance your skin then rinse off with warm water.

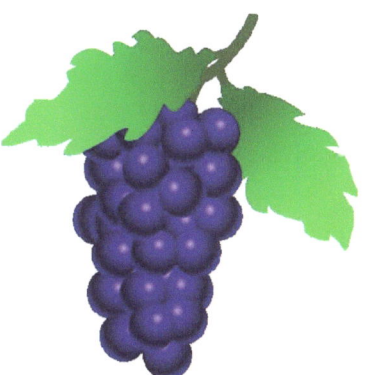

55. Grapes are rich in anti-oxidants, essential oils, vitamins and oligo-elements which are good in skin hydration and increasing blood circulation. Cut the grapes in halves then massage the juicy, and flesh parts over your face for 5 minutes. Leave the juice to dry the rinse off with warm water.

56. Use sweet almond oil to cleanse and soften the skin face; simply dab few drops of almond oil onto cotton ball then wipe makeup using almond.

57. Mix few drops of lemon juice with few drops of tea tree essential oil to half glass of distilled water and use cotton pads to apply the concoction to your face as a toner or a cleanser.

58. To get rid of blackheads, massage a generous fresh lemon juice onto your face. This will help in healing acne as lemon acts as antibacterial.

59. Shiny face? No worries, apply the lemon juice on your face to remove excess oil on your face.

60. Use chamomile tea to treat acne. Boil water and pour in a bowl and put the chamomile tea onto boiled water. Let it set for 3-5 minutes then use cotton ball to apply onto affected areas. Apply the tea twice a day on daily basis for at least 3 weeks in order to see the results.

61. Always wash your face after eating oily meals as the oils from the food can clog your pores.

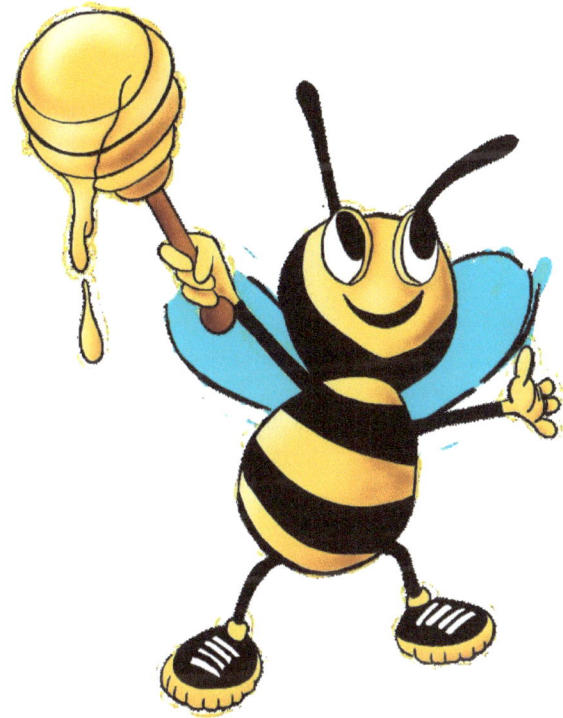

62. With its antibacterial properties, honey is great in removing any infectious substances that have the potential to clog the pores and cause zits. To stimulate your face, use honey as tonic. Simply pour 1-2 drops of honey onto damp palm and gently massage onto your face then pat dry.

63. Tea tree oil is good as an astringent to lessen redness, stinging and itching of the skin. It has antiseptic and antibacterial properties that help in getting rid of the bacteria that cause acne.

64. Pour tap water into a spray bottle and use it to spray on finished makeup. Hold the bottle 10 inches away from your face and spray, let the water dry naturally. This will leave your skin looking fresh, velvet and radiant and at the same time levelling out any foundation caught in fine lines.

65. For glowing skin and even skin tone, mix turmeric with lemon juice and apply the mixture to your face. Leave it on for 15-20 minutes then rinse well.

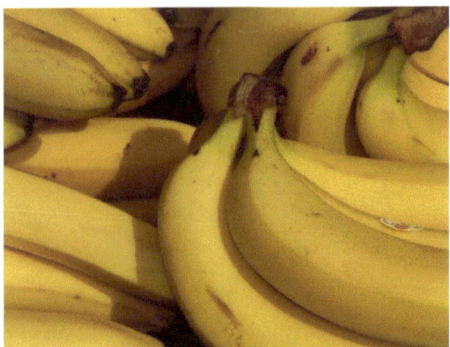

66. Mash a ripe banana and spread all over your face to cleanse it and reduce the appearance of wrinkles. Leave the mask on for 15-20 minutes then rinse it off with warm water followed by cold water. Gently pat dry your skin.

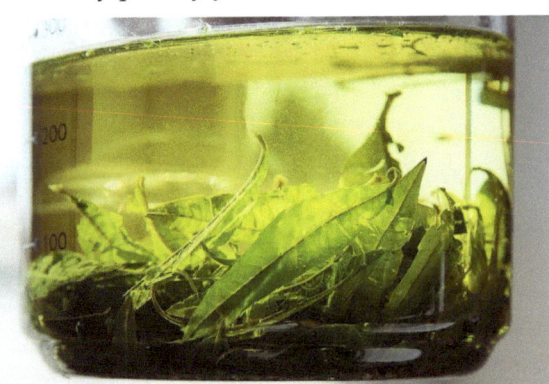

67. You can use green tea to remove blackheads. Simply mix 1 teaspoon of dry green tea leaves with water then scrub the mixture on the affected area. Leave it on for 3-5 minutes then wash it off with lukewarm water.

68. For oily skin, add 1 tablespoon of dried basil leaves to 1 cup of boiled water and soak them for 10 minutes. Strain the concoction and refrigerate until it cools then dab it on your face.

69. Use strawberries to reduce the swelling. Cut off the strawberry tops and use the fruit flesh to rub into your zits and leave for 25-30 minutes then rinse off.

70. To remove dead skin cells, use baking soda as an exfoliator. Simply mix small amount of soda with tap water then scrub the paste into your face then rinse well.

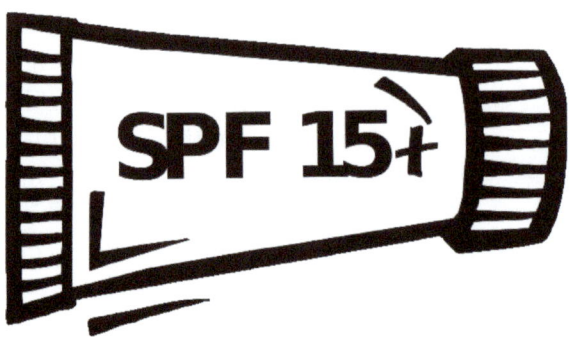

71. For oily face that is prone to blackheads, use oil-free make-up or sunscreens to avoid pore blockage and getting new blackheads.

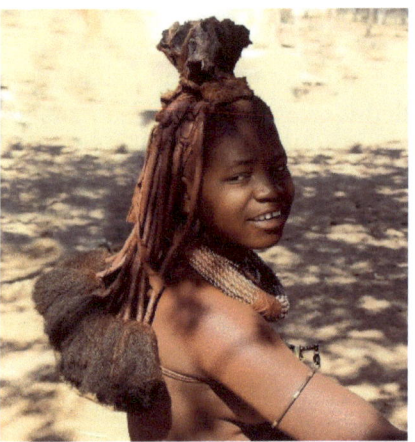

72. Ochre is a type of non-toxic iron oxide clay or sandy clay mineral found in natural deposits. African women have been known to apply the ochre powder in their faces as foundation and to beautify themselves. Ochre can assists with bad skin condition such as acne, reduce pigmentation and even-out the skin tone.

Hair and Scalp

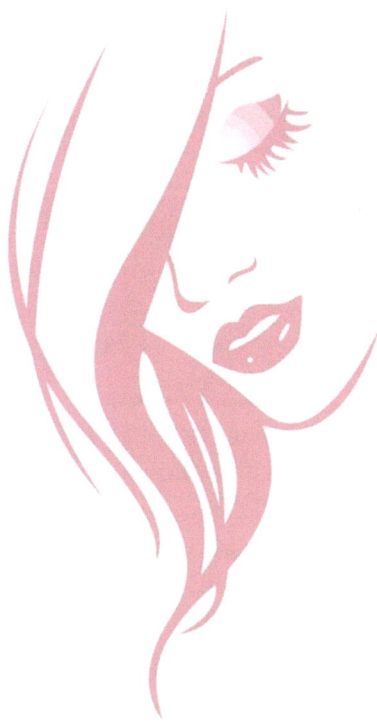

internal elements that affect their health status such as overexposure to invisible UV-B rays, pollution, extreme weather, harsh chemicals from hair care products, hormonal fluctuations and even the individual's diet and all these may result in thinning hair , damaged scalp (flaky or oily), dandruff and head lice breeding.

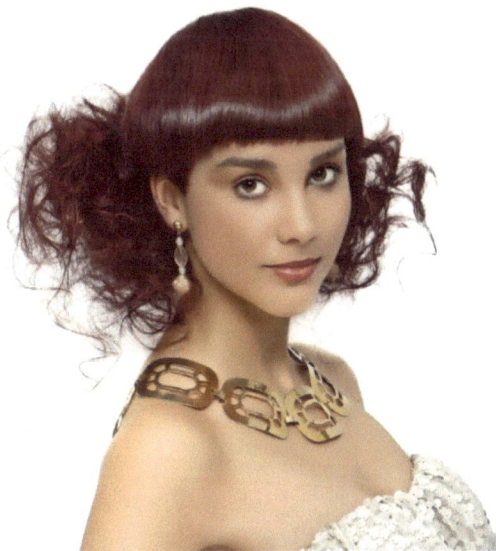

Hair has been used by many to express themselves through different hairstyles; hair is different in individuals and exhibits human diversity. The hair and the scalp can reveal the health conditions of an individual. Hair acts as temperature regulator and provides protection for the head. Hair care and scalp care intertwine as the scalp provides support for the hair and it is also responsible for producing oil which in turn develops a thin layer of protection for the hair roots.The sebaceous glands found in the scalp skin produce an oily substance known as sebum which is mainly made out of fatty acids. Sebum proves the hair with moisture and acts as protection against dryness; it inhibits microorganisms' growth and stops the hair from absorbing extreme quantity of external substances.

The hair and scalp are exposed to different, severe conditions and are susceptible to the effects of both external and

Cleaning and caring for the scalp ensures that the scalp is healthy and is not itchy and scaly. Whilst moderate sun rays are essential in assisting skin cells to produce vitamin D which helps in the biological process of hair repair, too much of the sunrays can leave the hair brittle and dry. To prevent bacterial infections and other scalp ailments, the scalp needs to be thoroughly cleansed to remove dead cells and toxin build-up from the scalp skin. Poor hygiene and diet can cause a great damage to the hair and scalp but most of these ailments are manageable and so put in place preventive measures such as cleaning of both the scalp and hair, eating healthy and regular scalp massage therapy to stimulate the blood vessels and nerves can assists in promoting healthy hair growth.

73. Spray your perfume onto your hairbrush before brushing your hair. The scent will stick to your hair's natural oils, giving it a subtle and appealing smell.

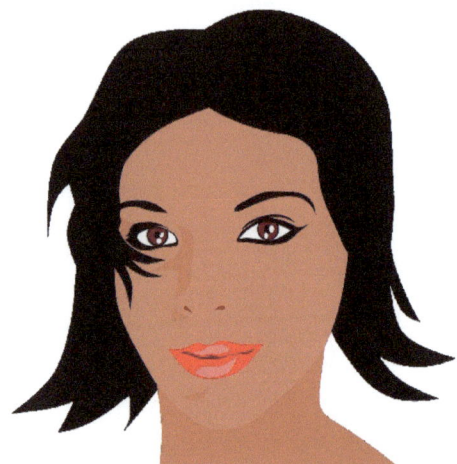

74. Massage your scalp every fortnight to help with hair growth and to stimulate your scalp's own natural oil production.

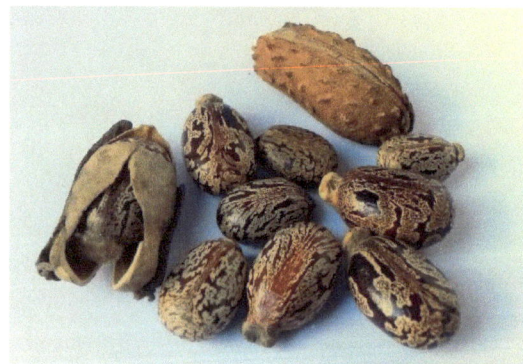

75. Mix 2 tablespoons of castor oil with 2 tablespoon of cognac. Apply the mixture onto your scalp onto and leave it on for 25-30 minutes then shampoo.

76. Use corn starch baby powder to shampoo your hair. Sprinkle a little amount in your hands, gently clap palms then rub them together and smoothly run them through the strands.

77. For glossy and nourished hair, rub in almond oil into your scalp and strands then leave it for 20-25 minutes before washing it.

78. Mayonnaise can be used for hair conditioning treatment and nourish your hair. Damp your hair with warm water. Apply mayonnaise to your hair then blow drying it to activate the amino acid known as L-cysteine and open the follicles, allowing the mayonnaise to enter the strands. Wrap your hair with shower cap to trap the heat and leave it on for 20 minutes or more. Rinse the mayonnaise off with warm water and let the hair to air dry. Shampoo your hair after 24 hours.

79. For radiant and glossy hair, apply mustard oil into your scalp and hair then cover your head with a shower cap. Use a hair dryer for 10-15 minutes to assist the oil to seep in then wash your hair and style however you want. Mustard oil is a source of fatty acids which assists in rejuvenating the scalp and stimulates blood circulation by making blood to move to the hair follicles.

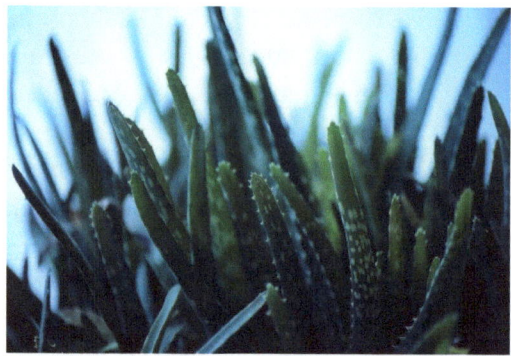

80. To assist your hair to grow, mix 2 tablespoons of aloe vera juice with 2 tablespoons of honey. Rub the mixture into your scalp and leave it on for 20 minutes then shampoo.

81. Purify your shampoo by adding a small amount of baking soda into your shampoo; this will prevent shampoo residue accumulation on your scalp.

82. To avoid your hair from tangling when washing, rub only in one direction.

83. To get rid of any dead skin left on the scalp after conditioning, rinse your hair with water mixed with few drops of apple cider vinegar.

84. Mix 1 tablespoon of mustard, 1 tablespoon of mayonnaise and a pinch of cayenne pepper and stir until all ingredients have blended. Apply the mixture onto your scalp and leave it on for 30 minutes then rinse with warm water and shampoo.

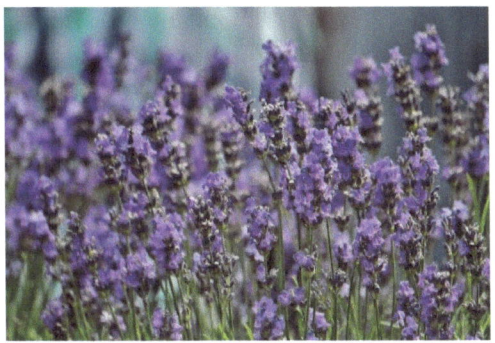

85. Lavender essential oil promotes hair growth by reviving its follicles, enhances hair quality and also gets rid of dandruff and lice. Mix 2 tablespoons of almond or olive oil with 15 drops of lavender essential oil then microwave the mixture until it is warm (not hot). Rub the concoction into your scalp, cover your head with shower cap and leave it on for 1 hour. Rinse with shampoo.

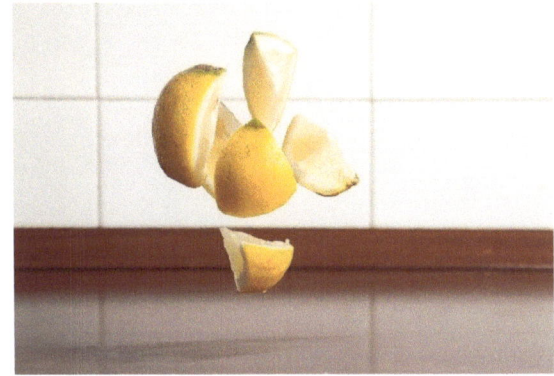

86. For dry scalp, apply lemon juice to your hair roots.

87. You can use coriander seeds to reduce hair loss and promote hair growth. Grind the coriander seeds until they turn into fine, smooth powder. Put 1 tablespoon of the powered into your regular hair oil and steep for a week. Apply the oil onto your scalp twice a week to revitalise your hair roots.

88. For greasy or oily hair, use either corn-starch or cornmeal to eliminate the grease or oil. Fill an empty and clean salt or pepper shaker with 1 tablespoon of corn-starch or cornmeal and sprinkle the whole content into the scalp and leave in for 10-15 minutes. Brush your hair with a paddle hairbrush by gently lifting hair at the roots and sweeping down.

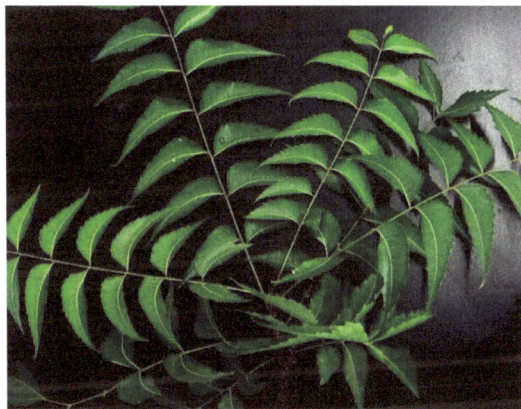

89. Use neem to get rid of dandruff. Boil a handful of neem leaves for half an hour; crush them until they turn into paste. Apply the paste into your scalp and leave it on for 30-35 minutes then rinse it off.

90. Use sour cream or plain yogurt to get rid of dirty on your hair. The milk fat found in these products moisturises the hair and the lactic acid in them clears any dirty coating in the hair. First damp your hair with water – take care not to make it too wet then rub in ½ cup of sour cream or plain yogurt and leave the product on the hair for 20-30 minutes. Rinse with warm

water then follow with a shampoo. Repeat the remedy every fortnight.

91. To treat dandruff and dry scalp, massage tea tree oil onto your scalp.

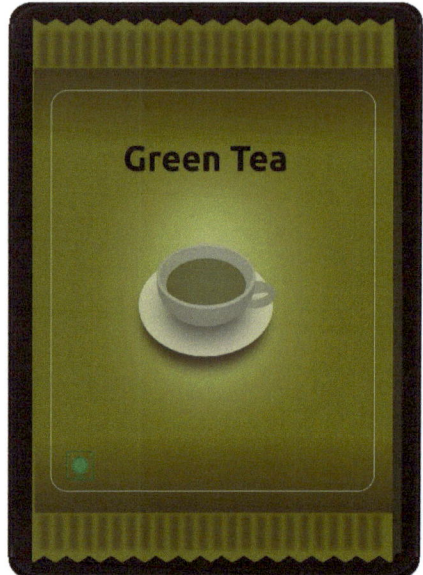

92. Green tea is concentrated with vitamin E, vitamin C and panthenol which are good at promoting hair growth, ease inflammation, strengthens hair and get rid of dandruff. Soak 4 green tea bags in 1 litre of boiling water and leave it to brew for 1 hour. After shampooing and conditioning your hair, rinse it with the fluid to achieve strong and glossy hair.

93. Apply lemon juice to your hair roots to remove dandruff.

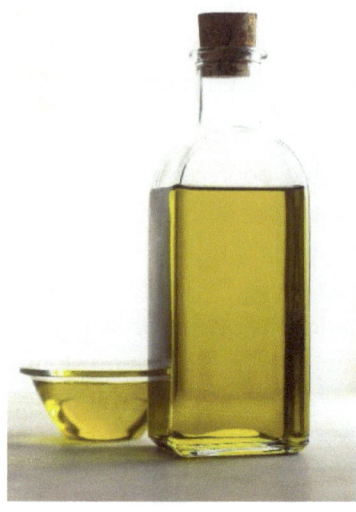

94. Use olive oil as a deep conditioning treatment to help in making the hair silk and enhance hair strength. Rub olive oil to your scalp so that your roots can absorb healthful fats and nutrients, leave it for 10-15 minutes and then wash it off.

95. For hair loss treatment, boil mustard oil and add some henna leaves to the simmering oil and let them burn in oil to absorb their minerals. Let the mixture cool then filter it with a fine strainer of thin cloth and massage your hair with the mixture daily.

Skin

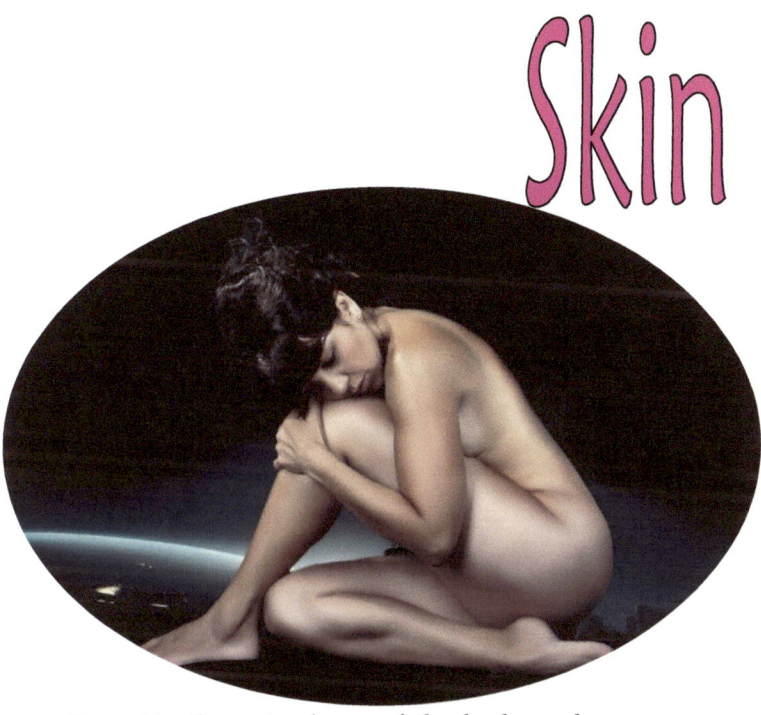

Our skin the outer layer of the body and its cells produce adequate amount of melanin to defend us from excess sun radiation and as such it needs to be protected. The skin is prone to all types of problems such as cellulite, sunburns, wrinkles and other infections.

Proper skincare means knowing one's skin type as it is crucial in knowing what best and what is not for one's skin. Your skin may fall under one of the following categories: normal skin, oily skin, dry skin, sensitive skin or combination skin.

Normal skin: This skin type is even toned with fairly visible pores. It has excellent elasticity and good balanced moisture and oil. Normal skin is usually healthy and smooth.

Oily skin: The skin usually looks oily and shiny and is prone to blackheads and acne due to the large pores and the skin producing excess oil and as such it is not able to get rid of dead skin cells that block the pores.

Dry skin: The skin has small pores and produces insufficient amount of oil which leaves the skin rigid, flaky and delicate. Dry skin prone to fine lines and wrinkles.

Sensitive skin: Although the skin can produce the right amount of sedum, it remains the most delicate skin type. The skin is vulnerable to even minor conditions and tends to bruise and burn easily and it is susceptible to pain and discolouring.

Combination skin: The T-zone which consists of the forehead, nose and chin of individuals with combination skin are usually dry while the other areas are oily.

Unlike other skin types, the combination skin requires prolonged beauty routine for both the treatment for oily skin for oily areas and for dry skin for dry area such as the cheeks and the area around the eyes.

Your skin type, age and environmental factors detect how you take care of skin but there are fundamentals of skincare remedies and routines that will ensure that your skin stays radiant, glowing and healthy at all times such as drinking plenty of water to replenish all the liquid your body have lost and hydrate your skin, good and healthy diet that include lot of fruits and veggies, quitting smoking, enough sleep, applying sunscreen whenever you are outdoor, and frequent exercise.

It is also advisable to see a professional dermatologist if you have persisting skin ailment before purchasing over the counter remedies. Above everything else, our skins need to be nourished from the inside first before concentrating on the outside and so, it is advisable to eat right, rest well, and drink enough water.

96. Want your skin to glow and have a more even tone after fake tanning? Then use an unscented cooking spray to improve your skin tone and moisturise.

97. If you ever run out of body moisturiser, do not despair, use coconut milk instance. Leave the coconut milk container opened overnight in the fridge. Use the solidified butter as a body moisturiser on your skin to make it soft.

98. Sake helps in anti-ageing and detoxification due to its rich minerals and amino acids. Add a cup of pure sake in a hot bath for flawless skin.

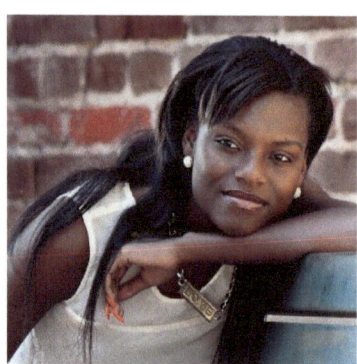

99. For glowing, agile and healthy skin, make a habit of using mustard oil paste. Mix equal amount of powered mustard seeds, turmeric powder, bedan (Bengal gram) and sandalwood with mustard oil. Put in 4 strands of saffron and massage the paste all over your body. Leave the paste on for approximately 20-30 minutes before taking a shower.

100. Use grape seed oil to remove stretch marks and heal scars.

101. Mustard oil can act as skin stress-reliever; it contains vitamin E which assists in hydrating the skin, detoxifying, improves blood circulation, reduces premature ageing, boosts skin quality and resistance. Massage the mustard oil on your skin daily.

102. How about a good bath of red wine? Pour red wine into your bath water to soothe and alleviate your skin.

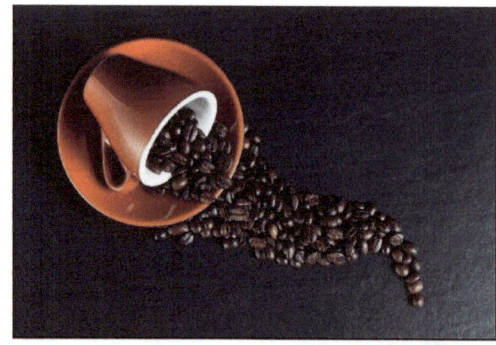

103. Caffeine can prove to be beneficial to your outer skin than to your inside. Use coffee grounds as a body scrub to stimulate your skin cells and remove dead skin. The caffeine in coffee helps to reduce the amount of fat cells and extract water making the cellulite to seem less obvious. Mix 2 tablespoon of extra-virgin olive oil with ½ cup of coffee grounds. Making sure the mixture sticks to the skin, massage the mixture to the affected areas then cover them with plastic wrap. Rinse with warm water after 10 minutes.

104. For young, velvety and healthy skin, take a bath of milk and honey mixed together. The alpha hydroxy acid and lactic found in milk helps in improving relaxation.

105. Free radicals are unstable cells which attack healthy cells in order to stabilise themselves. They can harm cells and are capable of fast-tracking the progression of age-related diseases, cardiovascular diseases and cancer. Grape seed oil assists in preserving ideal balanced elastin and collagen by reduce the effect of free radicals. Elastin is a protein found in connective tissues that allows body tissues to return to their shape after contracting or stretching and

collagen is a protein found in fibrous tissues and is crucial for strengthening blood vessels and provide the skin with elasticity and vitality. To attain flawless skin, use grape seed oil as a moisturiser.

106. The tannic acid found in black tea assists in healing sunburn by soothing the skin and lessening the burning feeling.

107. Grape seed oil has been reported to accelerate the treatment of wounds or broken skin as it accelerates restoration of skin tissues.

108. For radiant and glowing skin, splash ice cold water onto your face and breasts to increase blood circulation in these areas.

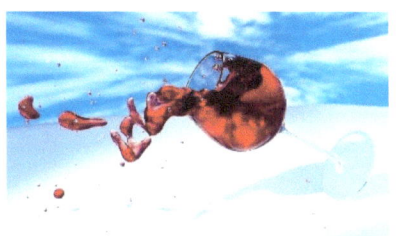

109. Drinking wine in moderation can assists in preventing heart diseases and protect against artery damage due to the presence of antioxidants in red wine called polyphenols.

110. Mix equal amount of jojoba oil, olive oil, series, and chamomile then place the mixture in ice tray overnight. Massage your face with the herb ice cube to refresh your face.

111. Use fresh tomato juice on your face to soothe and refresh your skin. Tomatoes contain lycopene, an anti-oxidant which offers soothing effects to your skin.

112. For oily skin, massage honey onto your skin to absorb excess oil while at the same time penetrating the skin to give it deep moisture it needs.

113. Use honey as anti-ageing skincare product and exfoliator. Honey consists of various excellent enzymes that get rid of dead skin cells and promotes the growth of new, healthier skin.

114. For supple skin, moisturise your skin within 3 minutes after cleansing to lock in moisture longer.

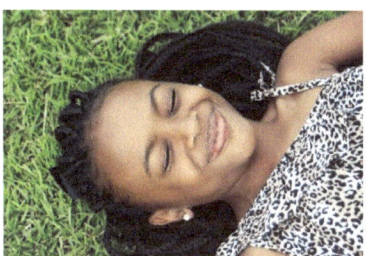

115. For clear and hydrated skin, mix lemon juice with coconut water and apply it as a moisturiser for flawless skin.

116. Always apply sunscreen even if the sun is not visible, including in winter time. Apply sunscreen onto your skin 30 minutes before going out and reapply it if you are exposed to the sun for more than 2 hours.

117. When scrubbing your skin, apply the scrubbing mixture in a circular motion all over your body, arms, thighs, legs, hands and feet. This helps in getting rid of dead skin cells and revealing glowing and healthy skin.

118. Grapeseed oil also contains fatty acids that are essential for robust and radiant skin and also contains linoleic acid which boosts skin wellbeing and assists build up cell membranes.

119. Mix 60 drops of one or two of essential oils to 120 ml of jojoba oil then massage the aromatic mixture to your skin daily for radiant and glowing skin.

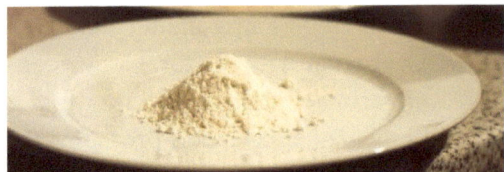

120. Mix turmeric with 1 gram of flour and water to create body scrub. Rub the paste all over your body before your shower or bath. This will give you a glowing and flawless skin in just weeks.

121. Green tea has properties that help in lessening inflammation and healing sun-burnt skin. Pour boiling water over green tea inside a bowl. Allow the tea to brew for 5 minutes and put it in the refrigerator to chill it. Submerge a cloth into the fluid and gently massage the affected area. Do not rub as this will only cause skin irritation.

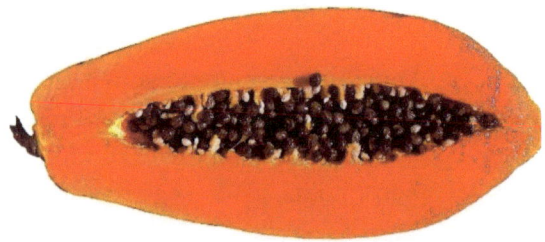

122. Papaya contains papain enzymes that good in exfoliating the skin. Simply peel the papaya, remove the seeds and pulverise the contents. Massage the paste onto your body and leave it on for 5-10 minutes then rinse it off in a shower.

123. Massage your wet body with dry salt after bath to exfoliate and improve blood circulation.

124. Use tamarind to exfoliate, promote circulation and to deep cleanse your skin. Mix 1 cup tamarind paste and 1 cup of honey with 4 cups of plain yoghurt. Using circular motions massage the cream onto your body and leave it on 5-10 minutes then rinse it off in a shower.

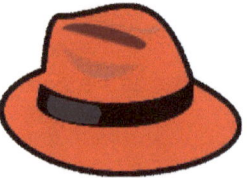

125. Cover your body by wearing sun blocking clothing when going outside for prolonged periods to protect your skin from overexposure to invisible UV-B rays.

126. You can use sesame oil to detoxify your skin. The sesame oil can get rid of toxins on the skin. Rub in warm sesame oil to your skin and leave it for 15-20 minutes then rinse it off with warm water without soap for optimum results.

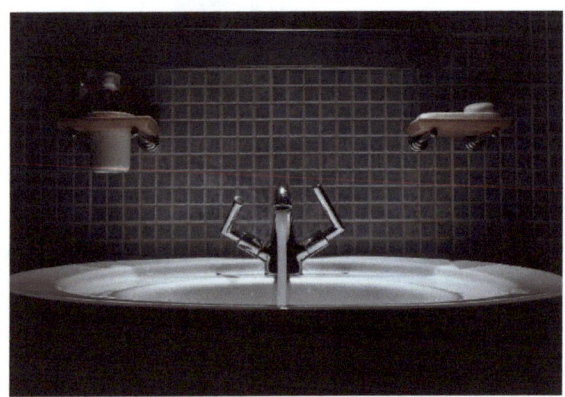

127. When bathing, keep the bathroom door closed to help keep the warm and steamy air. This will help to prevent your skin from drying up before moisturising it.

128. To treat itchy or burning skin and eczema, use rooibos tea bags. Brew a couple of rooibos tea bags in your bathwater and rinse the affected areas with the water.

Hands, Nails and Feet

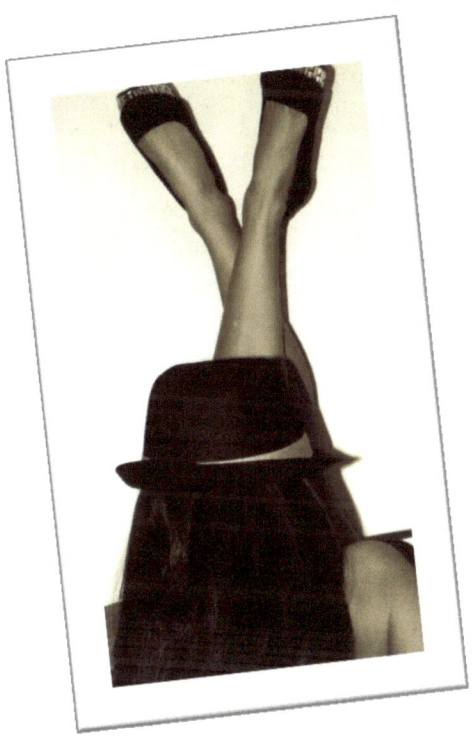

A proper nail care treatment includes a good care of the cuticles as most nail ailments start from there. Healthy and strong cuticles usually mean healthy and strong nails.

This is because the cuticles act as a protective shield for the tissues that are responsible for the growth of the nails. When the cuticles are not taken care of, they can tear and overlap the nails causing complications such as fungal nail infections like yeast infections, nail discoloration, abnormal nail shape, cuticle blisters, and soreness. Regular manicure ensures that the cuticles are smoothened out and pushed back as they can go.

Hands and Nails

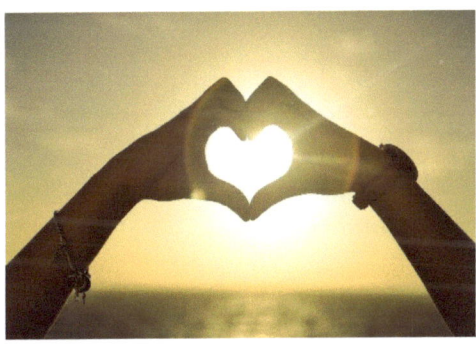

Our hands exposed to various elements because they act as our point of contact with lot of stuff such as opening doors, preparing food, handshakes and as such, they are exposed to germs all day long. Fingernails are made from keratin which is a protein which hardens as it ages. Nails protect our fingertips and are continuously growing and need to be trimmed constantly.

When it comes to cosmetic rituals, people often neglect their hands and nails the signs of pre-ageing such as wrinkles can start appearing in uncared for hands due to rupture of collagen and elastin. A good hand care routine is necessary to keep your hands young and soft; this includes moisturising them frequently throughout the day and before bedtime.

129. Mix few drops of olive oil, few coarse sea salt particles with water then scrub your hands with the mixture for at least 10 minutes. This will result in smooth hands.

130. For glossy nails, dab almond oil onto your nails every day.

131. To avoid nail polish from having bubbles when it dries after being applied on the nails, keep your nail polish in fridge, otherwise, always store your nail polish at cool temperature or room temperature.

132. For strong and shiny nails, eat almonds on an empty stomach to absorb their calcium.

133. Mix few drops of olive oil and lemon juice then soak your nails in the mixture to remove the yellow on the nails and also to strengthen brittle and dry nails.

134. Nail care should always be extended to the cuticles too. Mix baking soda with warm water and gently rub onto your cuticles.

135. Dip your fingertips in cold water for 3 minutes after manicure to dry the nail polish quickly.

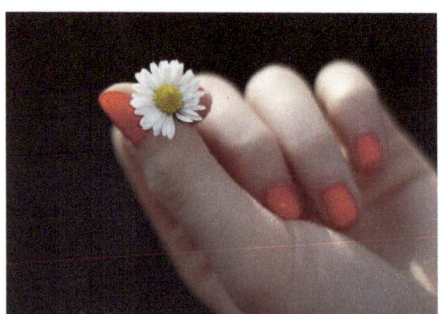

136. To make fragile, chipped nails use garlic. Chop a small fresh garlic clove and add it into a bottle of clear nail polish and let it sit for 5-7 days. Apply the mixture to your nails and the results will be shiny and stronger nails.

137. For soft hands, mix baking soda with warm water and gently rub onto your hands.

138. You can make your own hand cream that you can apply to moisturise and promote circulation on your hands. Mix 2/3 cup of rose water with 1/3 cup of glycerine and store it a bottle. Massage the cream in your hands frequently throughout the day.

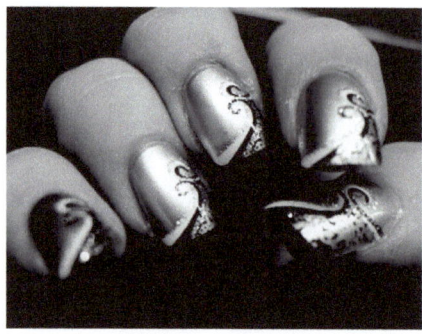

139. To remove glitter nail polish with ease, soak a cotton ball in a nail polish remover. Place it on the polished nail then wrap a tin foil around your finger and let it on for 5 minutes. The nail polish will glide away.

Feet

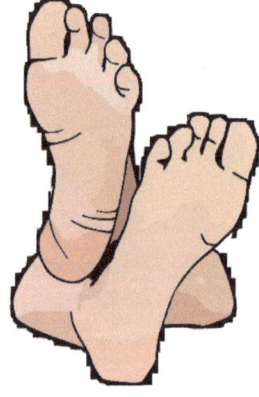

We spend most of time on our feet but sadly, these parts of our body receive little or no care at all. Foot wounds and injuries must be attended to immediately and people who live in warmer areas need to take extra special care of their feet to avoid athlete's foot which is a fungal or bacterial infection on the skin.

Here are some tips for keeping athlete's foot at bay:

- Replace synthetic socks with cotton socks which give the feet comfort and keep them dry.
- Apply fungicide powders between your toes to prevent bacterial spread and fungal growth.
- Wash your feet with medicated soap.
- Keep your feet and toes clean and moist free.

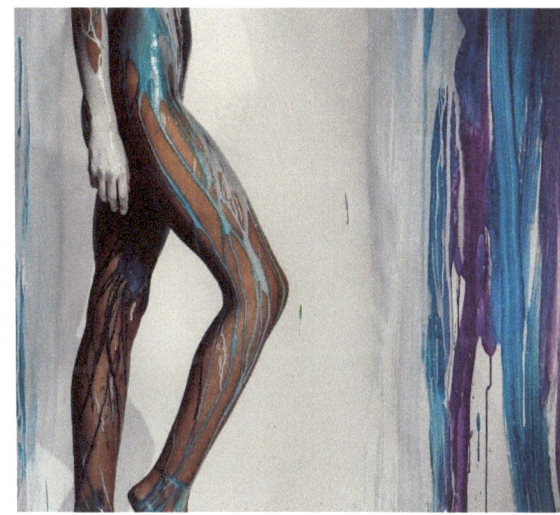

The skin on our feet need to be taken care of as it can be rough and calloused and simply running water over them is not enough, exfoliation by scrubbing them to remove dead cells and massage are essential to smooth and soft feet.

140. You can use red chili pepper to stimulate blood circulation and massage your feet. Pour hot water in a bowl and add dried red chili peppers then soak your feet for 10 minutes. Pat dry the feet then moisturise them.

141. To exfoliate your heels, rub the fleshy part of kiwi or pineapple skin onto the heels for 5-10 minutes then rinse off with warm water and pat dry. Moisturise the feet immediately to keep the moist.

142. To assists in repairing and hydrating cracked feet and elbows, apply diaper rash cream to your skin. The anti-inflammatory and moisturising properties of diaper rash cream speed the healing of the dehydrated and dry skin.

143. Tea tree essential oil has antibacterial property that can assists in treating athlete's foot. Apply the oil after taking a bath and before going to bed.

144. To treat athlete's foot, rub a pinch of baking soda between your toes and let it dry then wash your feet with clean, warm water.

Body

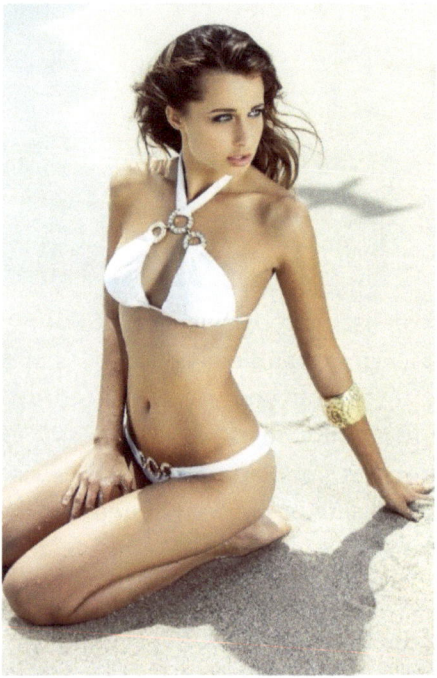

The human body contains about 75 trillion cells that are constantly working to keep us active and alive. These cells are constantly being renewed and replaced but their shape and characteristics stay constant throughout their lifespan. One of the unique things about our bodies is that no two bodies are identical and that make each one of us unique.

As much as our bodies can easily adapt to harsh conditions and experience constant process of renewing of cells and other body organs, we need to continuously take care of them in order for them to serve us well. Our daily habits detect our health conditions; a healthy body can be achieved by simply eating healthy and well-resting our bodies and exercising or performing physical activities for at least half an hour daily.

145. Avoid touching your face unnecessarily as this can cause pimple breakouts.

146. Need moisturiser that will not clog your pores? Massage pure almond oil onto your body every night.

147. Immerse 3 tablespoon of dried hibiscus into 2 cups of water, add honey and enjoy your tea.

148. Coconut oil contains lauric acid which assists in boosting metabolism, body cleansing, keeping bacterial infections at bay and also defends against cancers. Replace your cooking oil and Greek salad dressing with coconut oil. The coconut oil should be consumed not in excess.

149. Mix equal parts of baking soda with sea salt and add any essential oil. Pour the mixture to your bath for detoxification.

150. Now and then, we need to get a break from commercialised deodorant. Mix baking soda with water then apply the mixture on your armpits to stop body odour and sweat stains.

151. If you ever run out of shaving cream, use your hair conditioner to damp the area you want to shave.

152. Apply coconut oil before shaving your legs for nutritious hydration.

153. Squeezing zits damages tissues and also leave scars and as such avoid squeezing them.

154. To soothe out chronic inflammation of the skin and irritating, itchy and painful skin problems such as rashes, take 15-20 minutes long bath filled with rice twice a day.

155. Rice water has high concentration of carbohydrates and 8 essential amino acids and is good for drinking. These properties help in supplying your body

with energy and develop the building block for muscle and tissue renewing and revitalising respectively.

156. Make it a habit to include fruits and vegetables in your diet as they are nutritive and therefore assist in boosting your digestive system and also give you a healthy and glowing skin. Eat at least 5-7 portions of fruits and vegetables daily.

157. To improve your digestive system and bowel movement, eat organic foods as they contain probiotics which assists in aiding digestion.

158. To get rid of stomach gas, take 10-12 fresh mint leaves and chew them immediately after your meals. For better taste, put a pinch of candy sugar.

159. To avoid bloating, eat raw ginger before your meals. Cut a very thin slice of ginger and put a pinch of black salt on top of it then chew it slowly.

160. You can use turmeric to treat minor burns and cuts due to its antiseptic properties. Simply apply turmeric to the wound to ease the swelling.

161. To cure excessive menstrual bleeding use the devil's horsewhip (prickly chaff flower). Boil 1 tablespoon of powdered roots of the devil's horsewhip and drink the concoction twice a day.

162. Use unscented soap to wash the private parts and eat plain yogurt daily to get rid of unpleasant vaginal smell. You can also add the following to bathwater:

- Mix 10 drops of tea tree oil per litre of water
- Squeeze and mix the juice from 2-3 lemons per litre of water
- Mix 3-4 tablespoons of vinegar

163. Sleep can assists in good memory, it affects both physical and mental health. It is important for your well-being. Aim to have adequate sleep which ideally is 7-8 hours a night.

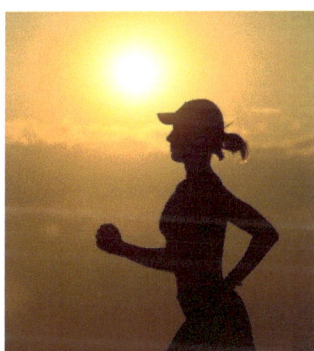

164. Exercise regularly. Exercise increases energy, fights diseases and health ailments, enhances mood and controls weight. Target at least 45 minutes of exercise or physical activity daily.

Weight Loss

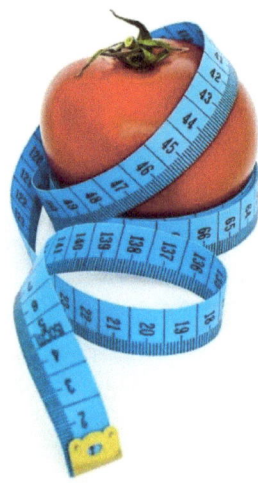

The journey to losing weight should be enjoyable and not frustrating as this can lead to binge eating for some people who see food as comfort zone. Some of the tips for people who want to lose weight and weight watchers:

- Minimise your intake of carbohydrates-rich foods, sweets and candies, refined sugars, red meat, excess salt, butter or ghee, oily, fatty and spicy foods.
- Avoid or stop smoking and overindulging in alcoholic beverages.

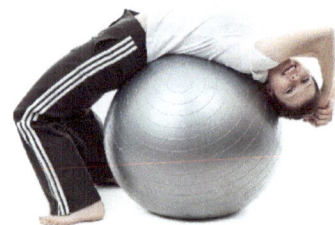

- Be physically active;
- Reduce your stress level and try to be positive and optimistic.
- Include green salad in one of meals on daily basis.

Good body image goes hand-in-hand with self-confidence and as such we need to love ourselves regardless of our body shape or weight. In order to kick-start a good weight loss or maintenance program, one needs to appreciate their body first. It is advisable to avoid fad food-starving diets that only bounce back as the users usual gain back the pounds they lost rapidly.

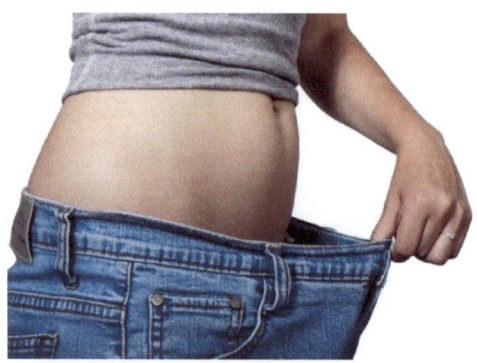

Losing weight in a healthy way may take time but it is good as the individual gain positive perspective and learns to feed their body in a healthy way. Try to focus on small steps instead of the end result and it will be easy to develop new, self-loving habits that can improve your outlook on life.

165. Water is one of nature's best gift to losing weight. Make sure your daily water intake is eight 8-ounce glasses (about 1.9 litres). Water helps in replenishing lost liquids, reduces your hunger level, transport nutrients to your cells, flushes toxins out of our vital organs and prevents water retention. Drinking cold water burns more calories as the body tries to heat the water up to body temperature; it speeds up your metabolism and curbs your appetite.

166. Black soybeans have many health benefits which include fighting inflammation, building muscles, block fat, control hunger pangs, decrease low-density lipoprotein (LDL) cholesterol (bad cholesterol) and increase high-density lipoprotein (HDL) cholesterol (good cholesterol). They also assists in weight-loss as they contain high fibre, high in protein and low-carb and as such, they take a long time to digest therefore making you feel fuller for long period. To curb your appetite, eat a half-cup of black soybeans half an hour before meals. This helps in you consuming fewer calories a day.

167. Replace high calorie fruit juices with fibre-filled fruits such as orange or grapefruit which help in suppressing appetite.

168. Soybean cocoa flour

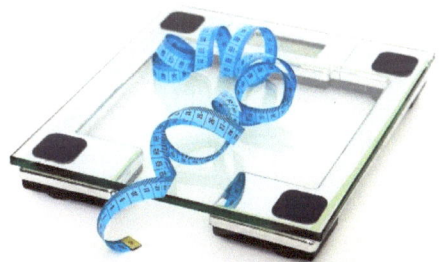

Want to lose weight without going on diet, then use black soybean flour cocoa.

Ingredients:
- 200 grams of black soybeans
- 100 grams of cocoa powder
- Milk
- Honey (you can substitute it with low calorie sweetener)

Process:
1) Wash the soybeans and drain out the water.
2) Roast the beans in a frying pan.
3) Use ladle to shuffle the beans while roasting until the beans start to split to reveal the whiteness inside then remove from the heat.
4) Put the beans in a household kitchen grinder and grind them until they are in powder form.
5) Mix the bean flour with the cocoa powder until they blend. Mix 20 grams of the soybean cocoa flour with 200 ml of warm milk.
6) Add honey or low-calorie sweetener for taste.

Store the mixture in an airtight container and put in the refrigerator. Take the mixture daily three times a day before meals to lose weight and control your craving for sweet things and hunger pangs.

169. Always keep your body hydrated at all times. Start your day with a glassful of water and end it with the same; have a glass of water when you wake up and other before getting in your bed. Drink a glass or two glasses of water before meals. Water fills your stomach up and therefore reducing your food intake. This helps the skin to glow, flushes out toxins from your body and keeps your appetite under control.

170. To reduce food craving and control your appetite, inhale grapefruit oil for 10-15 minutes. Always carry the oil with you in a small container.

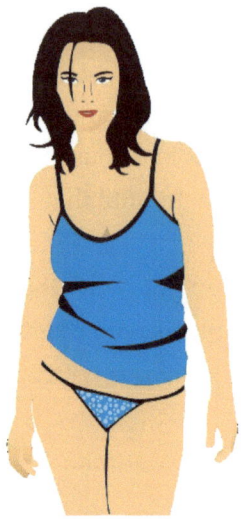

171. To reduce belly fat, mix 1 teaspoon of honey with 1 teaspoon of natural lemon juice into a glass of warm water and drink it daily 30 minutes before breakfast.

172. The enzymes found in vinegar can assists in getting rid of gas contents in your stomach by reducing the gastric juice production. To relieve the bloat effects, mix 1 tablespoon of apple cider vinegar with half a glass of water and drink the mixture. The mixture will start to de-bloat your system within 30 minutes.

173. Have you ever realised that the more sugar you consume the more you want to eat? That is because, sugar reduces the amount of the hormone that controls your hunger pangs and metabolism known as leptin and this results in slow metabolism and food cravings. Try and eliminate refined sugar from your diet.

174. When cooking, substitute oils such as vegetable oil, margarine or soybean oils with virgin olive oil, sunflower oil, sesame oil and virgin coconut oil as the former contain omega 6 fats that trigger heart diseases and hormonal imbalance.

175. Omega 3 fatty acids have been known for their properties to balance hormones and as such make sure you supplement them with vegan algae oil.

176. Reduce your caffeine intake as it slows down your thyroid. A thyroid is a ductless gland located in the neck. It is responsible for producing hormones that assist in controlling metabolism and growth.

General Tips

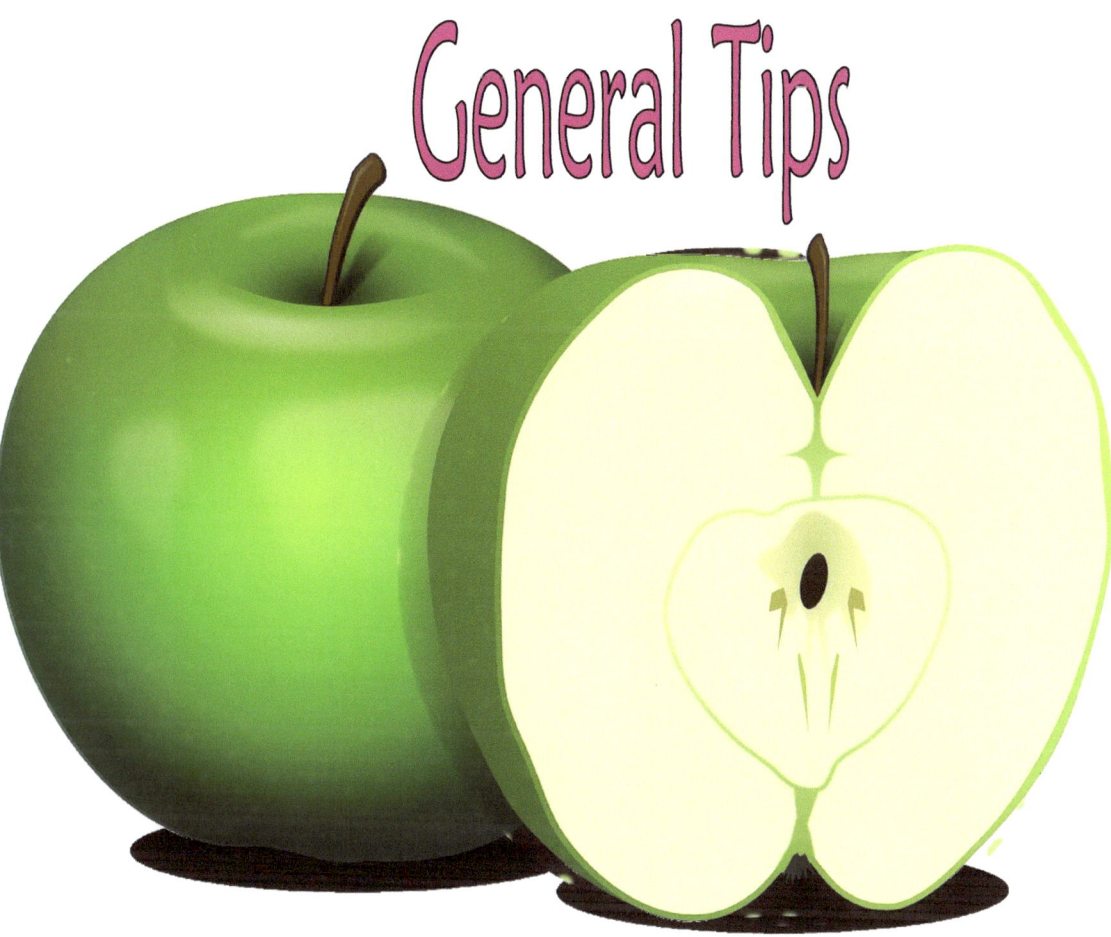

177. Popeye knew what he was doing when he gulped down can-full of spinach. Spinach contains phytonutrients that assists in detoxification and biotransformation system in the body. Wash raw spinach leaves, remove the spirals then put the green leaves in a juice maker. Drink the spinach juice twice a week for dazzling and radiant skin.

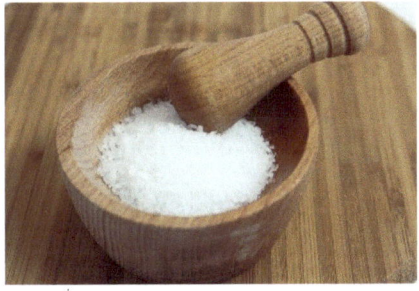

178. To keep aging at bay, try the ancient Greek secret, simply put about 1 gram of organic salt grains on the tip of your tongue after the meal. When the salt has dissolved, swallow the saliva.

179. To boost your mood and energy, use the dry rose hips. Mix equal parts of dry rose hips, nettles, knotweed and chopped dry grass and pour 1 tablespoon of the concoction in a cup of boiling water. Leave it to set for 3 hours then drink in one gulp. Replace your morning and afternoon tea intake with this blend.

180. Cut down on your intake of spicy food, sugared candy, cakes, refined flour and red meat in order to reduce body odour.

181. Drink a teaspoon of apple cider vinegar to stop hiccups.

182. Rinse your mouth with water mixed with small quantity of salt repeatedly throughout the day to cure mouth infections such as mouth sores, boils and cankers or gargle to relive sore throat.

183. Mix 1 teaspoon of salt with 1 teaspoon of baking soda in water and rinse your mouth with the mixture to get rid of bad smell.

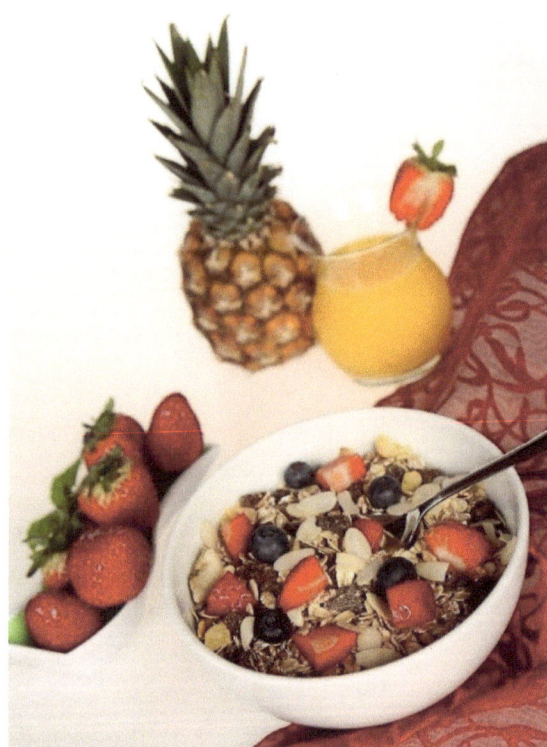

184. Make it a habit to start your mornings with regular, balanced breakfast. Breakfast forms an essential part of our healthy lifestyle and they keep our minds energised and alert.

185. To extend your toothbrush life, soak it in water mixed with salt before first use.

186. If you don't have appetite, have a lemon drink or eat sour snack to bring back your desire for food.

187. Out of mouthwash? Mix few drops of apple cider vinegar with water and swishes about the mouth to freshen your breath.

188. Slice a lemon with salt and pepper and suck on it to stop cough attacks.

189. Mix 1 tablespoon of baking soda in half a glass of water and drink it up to cure acid reflux.

190. To prevent bad breath when you are in between brushing, snack on some apples or any crunchy raw fruits or vegetables such as carrots. Apples boost salivary flow and as such cleaning inter-dental space.

191. Apply lemon essential oil to infections to assist them to heal more quickly.

192. To alleviate skin irritation, itchiness, mosquito bites place a poultice of salt mixed with olive oil on the affected part.

193. Almonds are good source of calcium and they produce alkaline which is good at balancing your body pH. To alleviate acid reflux, eat raw almonds.

194. If you suffer from constant acid reflux or if you want to minimise your chance of having it, drink about 60 ml (2 oz.) of unprocessed aloe vera juice daily.

195. If you are feeling restless and cannot fall asleep at night, try counting 100 sheep but rather than counting them the normal way, try counting backward. For this technique to be successful, try to stay calm and avoid getting annoyed with yourself and count slowly and whenever you get lost, start all over again. This activity will prove to be monotonous to your brains and cause you to sleep.

196. To relieve wet cough, mix 2 tablespoon of honey with 1 teaspoon of freshly ground pepper and boiled water. Honey acts a cough alleviator while the pepper

accelerates circulation and mucus flow. Allow the mixture to soak in (steep) for 15 minutes, strain then drink.

197. Use apple vinegar to prevent the breeding of odour-producing bacteria. Simply apply the apple vinegar in your armpits.

198. Practise correct breathing technique (CBT). The CBT assists in reducing stress levels, helps in relaxing your body in returning enabling you to sleep better, improves concentration, through exhaling the body gets rid of carbon dioxide, the toxin that is produced by the body and oxygen gets into the body through inhaling. Oxygen helps the body to function more efficiently and improves the digestive system functioning. This is how to perform CBT:

   a. Close your mouth then inhale air through your nose and counting to four then breathe out after a couple of seconds.

   b. Now slowly exhale the air through your mouth whilst counting to ten.

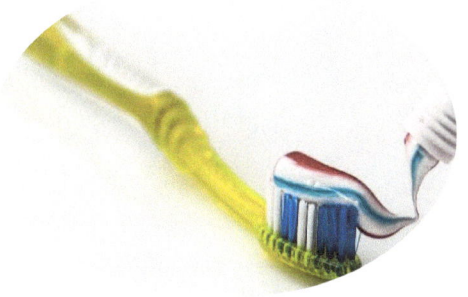

199. If you ever run out of toothpaste, don't despair, mix 1 part of fine salt with 2 parts of baking soda.

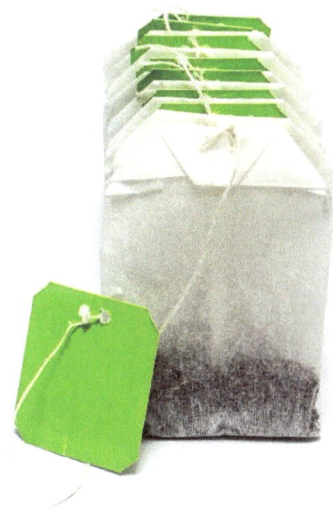

200. Green tea and rooibos tea are rich in unique blends of antioxidants, amino acids and minerals. Rooibos assists in deactivating and restricting the production of free radicals before they can cause any damage. Rooibos can be used to treat allergy symptoms such as hay fever and runny noses. Simply cup lukewarm water rooibos tea in your hands and slowly pull in the tea into your sinuses. Hold the liquid in for a few seconds then release it. Blow your nose gently.

201. Apple cider vinegar has antibiotic properties that assist in easing diarrhoea caused by bacterial infection and it also contains pectin that assists in pacifying intestinal spasms. Mix 1-2 tablespoons of apple cider vinegar with water then take the mixture.

Homemade Body Scrubs, Bubble Baths and Perfumes

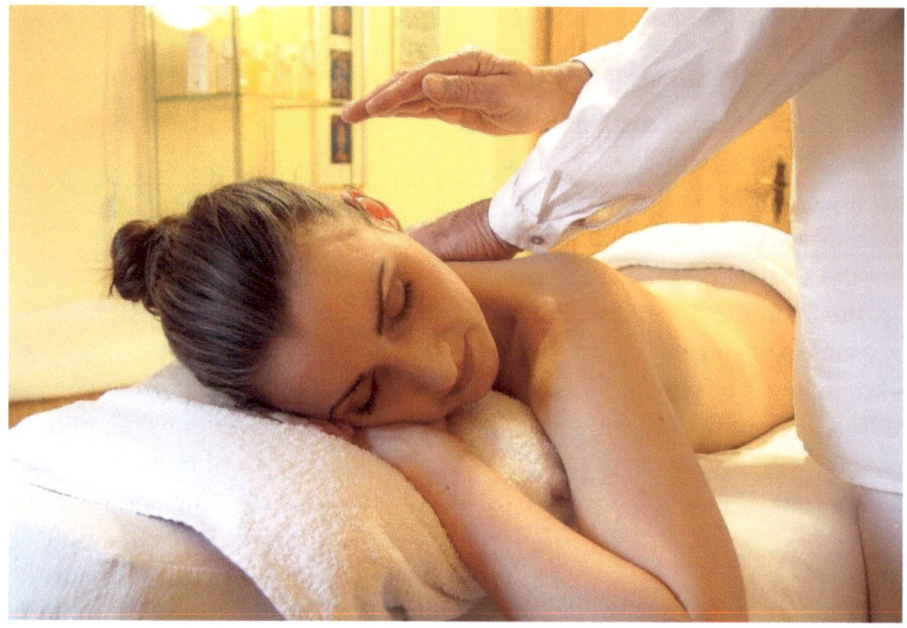

Our bodies need to be pampered every now and then; you do not need to pay through your nose to do just that. You can have your own affordable, cheap and yet quality spa treatment at home. At any given time, our homes are fully-equipped with most if not all of ingredients needed to make homemade body scrub recipes, so why not make use of them and indulge your skin, after all, it deserve it, don't you think? Taking care of your skin can reduce the signs of ageing and blemishes. Below are some of benefits of using homemade body scrubs:

- They exfoliate the skin and therefore getting rid of old layers of dead skin and leaving the pores unclogged.
- They promote skin regeneration and leave the skin healthy, fresh, smooth and glowing.
- They are cheap and easy to make.

1. Coffee Ground Mask

To get unblemished and glossy skin, mix 4 parts coffee grounds to 4 parts olive oil and 1 part lemon juice and apply the concoction to your skin.

2. Body Cream

Mix ½ cup of lanolin, ½ cup of castor oil and ½ cup of glycerine. Melt the mixture on a very low heat while gentle stirring. Let the cream cool then store in a jar and apply when needed.

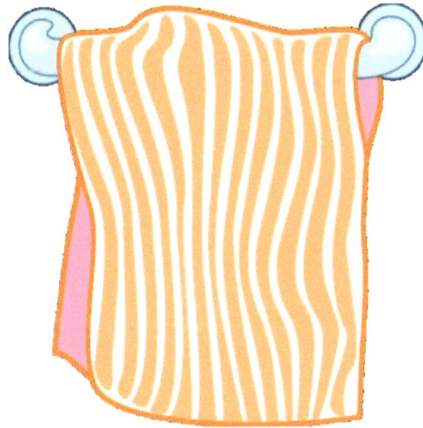

3. Whipped Coconut Body Butter

Ingredients:

- 1 cup of solidified coconut oil
- 10-15 drops of myrrh or any essential oil of your choice

Process:

a. Pour the coconut oil into an electric mixer.
b. Whip at high speed for 5 minutes or until the oil turn to be fluffy and light and pour in a mixing bowl.
c. Add in myrrh or your preferred essential oil and mix well until the ingredients blend together.
d. Fill in the mixture into a jar and store in a cool place.
e. Use the body butter to moisturise your skin after every bath.

4. Essential Oil Scented Deodorant

Using essential oils to make deodorant does not only give you great smell, it also has beneficial features as most essential oils are therapeutic and can help to de-stress, relaxes and elevate your mood. Fractionated Coconut Oil is natural carrier oil that easily absorbs into the skin without clogging the pores and it is good for dry skin.

Ingredients:

- 1.5 teaspoon of fractionated coconut oil
- ½ teaspoon of jojoba oil
- 20 drops of grapefruit essential oil
- 15 drops of peppermint essential oil

Process:

a. Pour all ingredients into 10 ml deodorant bottle with a roller.
b. Shake well to blend the ingredients.

5. Honey Brown Sugar Body Scrub

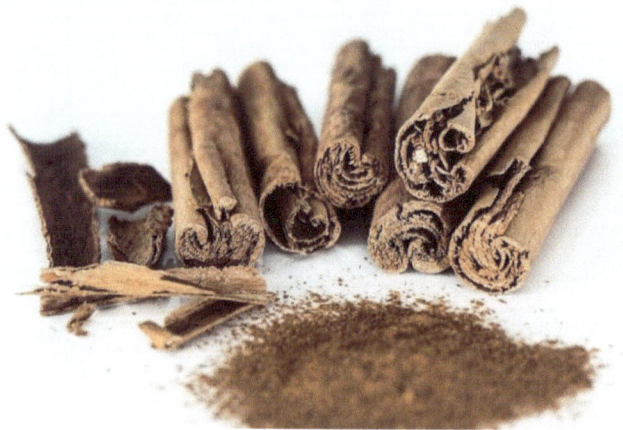

Ingredients:

- 2 cups of brown sugar
- ¼ cup of honey
- ½ cup of olive oil
- 1 teaspoon of vanilla
- ¼ teaspoon of cinnamon

Process:

a. Mix all the ingredients in a mixing bowl.
b. Empty the mixture in a jar and store in a cool place.

6. All Natural Solid Perfume

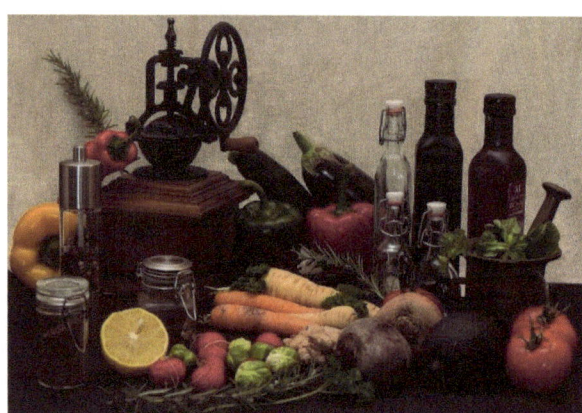

Ingredients:

- 3 parts of sweet almond oil or jojoba oil or olive oil (you are spoilt for choice)
- 1 part beeswax or substitute with soy wax
- Essential oils: the essential oils have different aromas that can change people's moods. Use the essential oils below to come up with your own personal fragrant:

- o **Citrus scents** include: grapefruit, lemon, lime and orange
- o **Floral scents** include: chamomile, Jasmine, Lavender, Rose and Ylang-ylang
- o **Herbal/ Fresh scents** include: Basil, Chamomile, Clary sage, Peppermint and Rosemary
- o **Camphor-like scents** include: Eucalyptus, Peppermint, Rosemary and Tea tree
- o **Spicy/Exotic scents** include: Aniseed, Black pepper, Cinnamon, Coriander, Ginger and Nutmeg
- o **Resinous balsamic scents** include: Frankincense and Myrrh
- o **Woody scents** include: cedar, Cinnamon, Pine and Sandalwood
- o **Earthy scents** include: Angelica and Patchouli

Process:

a. Mix the oil and beeswax or soy wax together in a microwave bowl and heat them in microwave until the wax melts or on a stove.

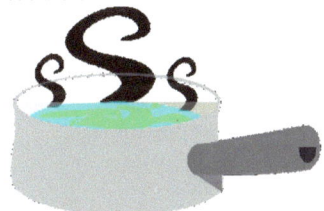

b. Remove the mixture from the heat. (If you are using the stove, pour the mixture in a mixing bowl.)
c. Add 10-15 drops of essential oils of your choice and stir well.
d. Pour the perfume into a jar and let it set for half an hour to an hour before using it.

7. **Eucalyptus Bubble Bath**

This cold relief bubble bath is good in easing cold, muscle aches, stuffy nose and congested chest. Soak in the cold relief bubble bath for at least 10 minutes. To get the most value of the essential oils, breathe deeply through the nose and exhale from the mouth.

Ingredients:

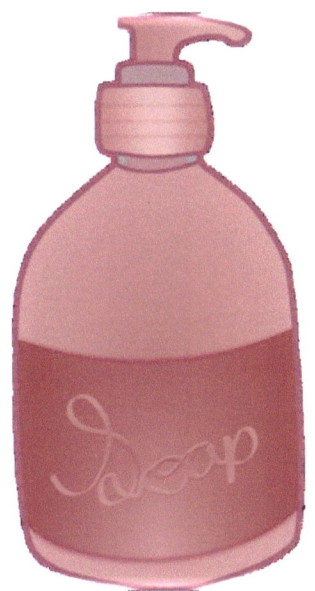

- 6 drops of eucalyptus essential oil
- 3 drops of peppermint essential oil
- 3 drops of spearmint essential oil
- 3 drops of grapefruit essential oil
- 1 quart distilled water
- 4 ounces castile soap bars
- 4 ounces glycerine

 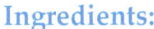

Process:

a. Mix the distilled water, castile soap and the glycerine together in bowl and stir them until they blend.
b. Add the eucalyptus essential oil, peppermint essential oil, spearmint essential oil and grapefruit essential oil to the mixture and blend you have a uniform concoction.
c. Store the bubble bath in a clean and re-sealable jar and use it in you baths.

8. Chamomile Bubble Bath

This bubble bath will leave your skin smooth, relaxed, soft and moisturised while reducing the appearance of wrinkles and fine lines. Always shake the bottle gently before pouring in bathing water.

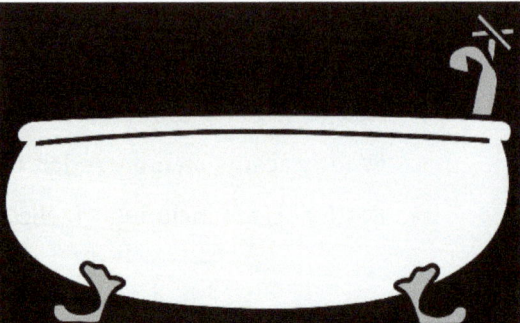

Ingredients:

- ½ cup of fresh dried chamomile
- 4 drops of vanilla essential oil
- 4 cups of powdered milk
- 1 quart distilled water
- ½ cup of unscented castile liquid soap

Process:

a. Boil the water then remove it from the heat.
b. Add chamomile to the water then close the pot with a tight, fitting lid. Let the herb steep for 25-30 minutes and then strain them.
c. Pour the mixture into a bowl then add the powdered milk, vanilla essential oil and the castile soap.
d. Mix the concoction until it blends and then store in airtight plastic bottle.

9. Tea Tree Essential Oil Vaginal Wash Remedy

Yeast infections, vaginal pH imbalance and a bacterial infection known as bacterial vaginosis can cause strong, unpleasant vaginal odour using scented soaps to wash the female genitalia as they change the required vital vaginal acidity and this can cause yeast infection. Tea tree oil is good at curing bacterial growth and fighting vaginal odour.

Ingredients:

- 3 drops of tea tree essential oil
- 1 cup of lukewarm water

Process:

a. Mix tea tree essential oil with the water and stir well.
b. Wash the vagina with the mixture.

10. Almond Oil Nourishing Cream for Dry Skin

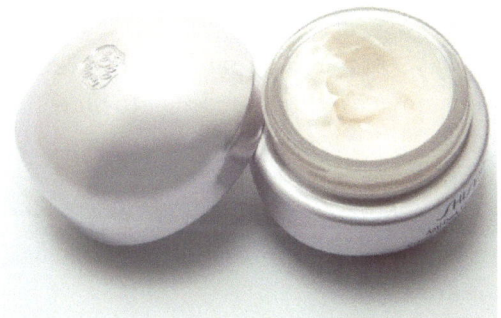

Use this cream to strengthen your skin cells and hydrate your dry skin.

Ingredients:

- 4 tablespoons of almond oil
- 1 tablespoon of beeswax
- 2 tablespoon of rose water

Process:

a. Mix all the ingredients and then store in airtight bottle.

11. Oatmeal, Chamomile and Rosemary Soap

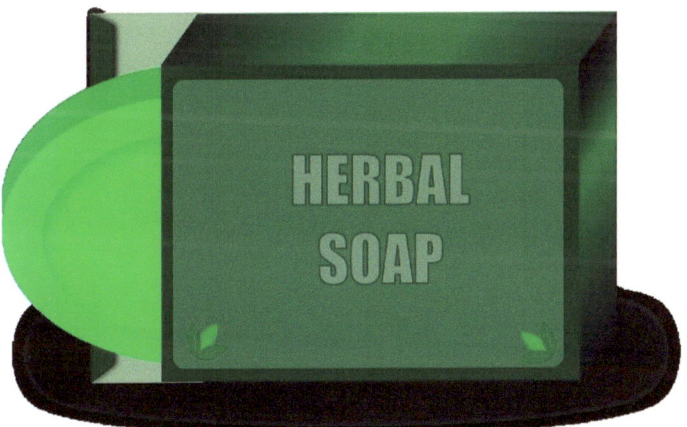

Ingredients:

- ¼ cup of dried rolled oats
- 120 ml of castile soap
- ¼ cup of distilled water
- 1 tablespoon dried Chamomile
- 1 tablespoon dried Rosemary
- 1 tablespoon Jojoba oil
- ½ tablespoon of vitamin E oil

Process:

a. Grind the oats in a food processor until powder.
b. Grate the castile soap.
c. Bring the distilled water to boil in a saucepan. Take off the saucepan from the heat.
d. Put the chamomile and rosemary into the water and leave the concoction to brew for 30 minutes.
e. Use a fine-sieve strainer to filter the water and dispose of the herbs.
f. Reheat the water over low heat until it boils.
g. Add the grated castile soap and mix until the concoction until it blends and becomes thick and glutinous. Remove the saucepan from the stove
h. Add the oats, jojoba oil and vitamin E oil and blend well.
i. Pour the mixture into a soap mould and let it set for at least 5 hours at room temperature.
j. When the soap solidified, remove it from the mould and use it for baths.

12. Feet Soak

Use this remedy to soften your feet before bedtime.

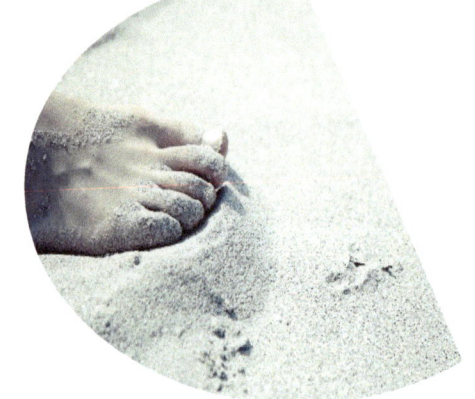

Ingredients:

- 4 cups of water
- 1 teaspoon of peppermint oil
- ¼ cup of sea salt

Process:

b. Boil the water.
c. Add the salt to the boiling water.
d. Leave the mixture to cool to your desirable warmth then add the peppermint oil.
e. Soak your feet in the remedy for 15-30 minutes then rinse them.

*** You can add 1 teaspoon of vitamin E oil to increase the life span of your body scrubs and make sure you store them in airtight containers.

Homemade Face Masks (Facials) & Other Remedies

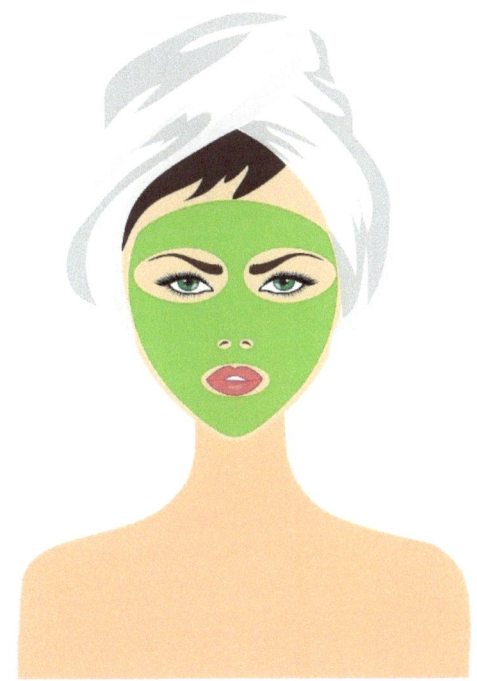

Facial masks offer many benefits to our facial skin, they:

- Promote and stimulate circulation and unclog the pores;
- Cleanse and help in conditioning and rejuvenating the skin which promote healthy skin and healing;
- Detoxify the skin by getting rid of dead skin cells and other dirt from the skin;
- Offer deep nourishment by replenish the skin with nutrients;
- Moisturise: they provide moisture to the skin which assists in hydrating the skin, reducing the effects of aging and dry skin.

One does not to go a spa to pamper themselves; rather you can add this much needed skincare routine to your already existing routines and without breaking the bank. You can make face masks from natural ingredients with antioxidant, emollient and soothing properties found in the kitchen or garden. Not only are homemade facial mask cheap, they also revive lifeless, aging and dull facial skin, regenerate skin cells, firm the skin and promotes excellent skin tone.

1. **Soy Milk Mask**

   To reduce pores use soy milk by soaking gauze in it and then apply it to your face then rinse it off an hour before bedtime.

2. **Nightingale Droppings Facial**

   Japanese women should be praised for having known the benefits of using nightingale droppings as exfoliator and moisturiser. Not only does the bird poop get rid of excess pigmentation, it also acts a skin lightening. Collect the droppings, sun-dry them then mix them with water and apply on your face for 15 minutes. If looking for bird poop is not amongst your to-do lists, you can purchase the UV-sterilised droppings powder in a local Japanese shop if it is available.

3. **Rice Bran Facial**

   The B-complex vitamins found in rice bran can help in stimulating blood circulation. Grind the rice bran until it is powdery then mix with water. Apply the cream into you face to scrub or leave it on for 15 minutes as a mask.

4. **Apple Juice Facial**

   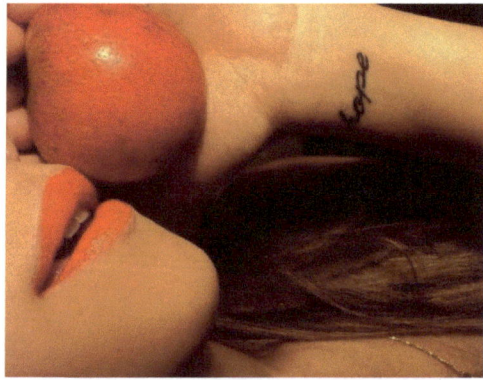

   Exfoliate your face with the mixture of apple juice, milk and egg white. Mix 3 tablespoons of apple juice with 3 tablespoons of milk and 1 egg white. Apply the mixture to your face and leave for 15-20 minutes then rinse with warm water.

5. **Mustard Oil and Lemon Juice Paste**

   Mix turmeric powder with mustard oil droplets and lemon juice then apply the mixture onto your zit and leave for 15 minutes. Gently scrub and wash your face with plain water. The remedy is effective if it repeated 2-3 times a week.

6. **Almond Cleansing Face Mask**

For soft skin, soak ½ of a cup of almonds overnight. Add a dash of saffron into the paste. In the morning, splash your face with clear, warm water then apply the thick cream onto your face and leave it on for 20-25 minutes. Moist your fingertips and gently scrub the dry paste in circular motions.

7. **Cinnamon and Honey Face Mask**

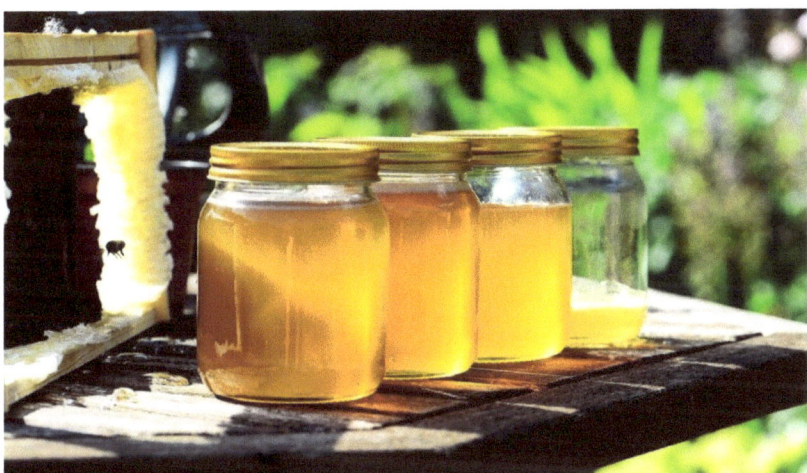

Mix ½ tablespoon of cinnamon with 1 tablespoon of honey. Apply the paste onto your face and leave it for 25-30 minutes.

8. **Sugar and Lemon Juice Facial**

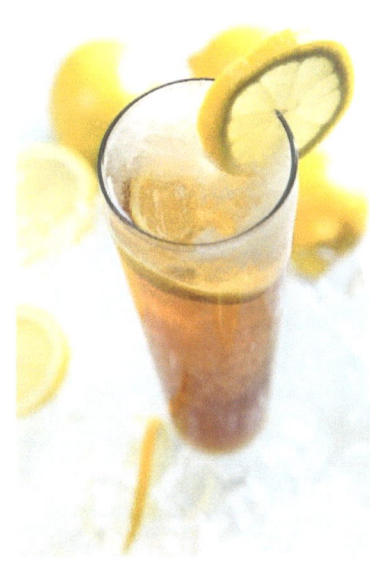

To eliminate blackheads and to control oil in your oily face, mix sugar with lemon juice to make paste. Rinse your face then apply your homemade exfoliator to your face in gentle, light and circular motions for 5 minutes. Rinse well with warm water.

9. **Nutmeg and Buttermilk Face Mask**

To get rid of blemish and reduce oil in your oily face, mix nutmeg with buttermilk cream to make paste. Rinse your face then apply your homemade exfoliator to your face in gentle, light and circular motions for 5 minutes. Rinse well with warm water.

10. Baking Soda Facial

For oily face, mix baking soda with water to make paste. Rinse your face then apply your homemade exfoliator to your face in gentle, light and circular motions for 5 minutes. Rinse well with warm water.

11. Sour Cream Mask

To reduce blackheads and to manage oil in an oily face, mix salt with sour cream to make paste. Rinse your face then apply your homemade exfoliator to your face in gentle, light and circular motions for 5 minutes. Rinse well with warm water.

12. Baking Soda Steam

Add 1 tablespoon of baking soda to a cup of distilled water. Apply the paste to your face. Bring a small pot of water to a boil. Hold your face over the steaming water with a towel draped over your head so that it creates a sort of tent over your face and help concentrate the steam. Keep your face over the steam for about 10 minutes. Wrap your fingers in cotton pad and gentle remove the paste from your face.

13. Cinnamon and Honey Face Mask

Mix 1 tablespoon of cinnamon powder and honey to create a thick paste. Apply the concoction to your face and leave it on overnight. Rinse it off in the morning. Use the remedy for 10 consecutive days to get rid and prevent blackheads.

14. Lemon Facial

To banish blackheads, use the lemon facial scrub. Mix lemon juice with salt, honey and yogurt then gently rub on the affected area.

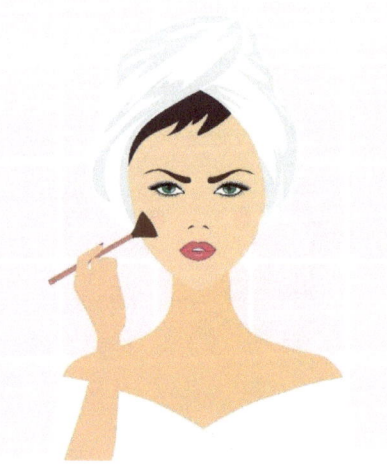

15. Turmeric and Sandalwood Facial

Mix turmeric with a small amount of sandalwood powder and water in a mixing bowl. Apply the paste onto your face to reduce acne.

16. Peppermint and Lemongrass Essential Oils Face Steam

The aromas from peppermint and lemongrass essential oils can assist in energising you.

Process:

a. Pour hot water into a small bowl.

b. Add 3 drops of peppermint or lemongrass essential oil then hold your face 30 cm (about 12 inches) above the bowl and over the steaming water with a towel draped over your head so that it creates a sort of tent over your face and helps concentrate the steam.

c. Keep your face with your eyes shut over the steam for about 5 minutes. If the steam gets too much, raise the towel to let in fresh air then resume the therapy.

17. Lavender/Chamomile Essential Oil Face Steam

Use lavender or chamomile essential oil to relax your mind.

Process:

a. Pour hot water into a small bowl.

b. Add 3 drops of lavender or chamomile essential oil then hold your face 30 cm (about 12 inches) above the bowl and over the steaming water with a towel draped over your head so that it creates a sort of tent over your face and helps concentrate the steam.

c. Keep your face with your eyes shut over the steam for about 5 minutes. If the steam gets too much, raise the towel to let in fresh air then resume the therapy.

18. Eucalyptus Essential Oil Face Steam

Eucalyptus essential oil is good in getting rid of cold symptoms.

Process:

a. Pour hot water into a small bowl.

b. Add 3 drops of eucalyptus oil then hold your face 30 cm (about 12 inches) above the bowl and over the steaming water with a towel draped over your head so that it creates a sort of tent over your face and helps concentrate the steam.

c. Keep your face with your eyes shut over the steam for about 5 minutes. If the steam gets too much, raise the towel to let in fresh air then resume the therapy.

19. Bergamot/Sandalwood Essential Oil Face Steam

If you feel stressed-out, use bergamot or sandalwood essential oil to uplift your mood.

Process:

a. Pour hot water into a small bowl.

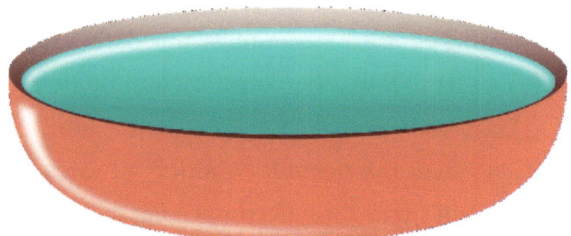

b. Add 3 drops of bergamot or sandalwood oil then hold your face 30 cm (about 12 inches) above the bowl and over the steaming water with a towel draped over your head so that it creates a sort of tent over your face and helps concentrate the steam.

c. Keep your face with your eyes shut over the steam for about 5 minutes. If the steam gets too much, raise the towel to let in fresh air then resume the therapy.

20. Turmeric and Sugarcane Facial Juice

Get rid of wrinkles by using turmeric. Mix a small amount of turmeric with sugarcane juice and apply the paste to your face.

21. Sweet Potato and Carrot Face Mask

To encourage circulation, reduce skin ageing and loosen up your facial muscles, use the vegetable facial mask during winter time.

Ingredients:

- 1 medium carrot
- 1 small sweet potato
- 1 large egg yolk
- 2 tablespoon of milk

Process:

a. Steam the carrot and sweet potato.
b. Peel the steamed veggies and mash them together in a bowl.
c. Add in the egg yolk and milk to the mixture and blend the ingredients until they turn into uniform thick paste.
d. Rub on a generous coat of the warm paste onto your face and leave it on for 15-20 minutes. Rinse with warm water.

22. To alleviate athlete's foot, use vinegar as a remedy. Mix 10-15 drops of vinegar into half bucket of water and soak your feet in the mixture.

23. Mix 2-3 tablespoon of salt in ½ bucket of warm water and soak your feet in the mixture to get rid of fungus between the toes.

24. Pineapple and Apple toner

To heal a broken skin and reduce the appearance of fine wrinkles on your face use this remedy.

Ingredients:

- 1 medium green pineapple
- 1 large apple

Process:

a. Use the juicer to extract the juices from the fruits.
b. Apply the concoction to your face and leave it on for 10-15 minutes.
c. Rinse off with clean, warm water.

25. Syrup tonic

This tonic assists in fighting fatigue and leaves you feeling invigorated.

Ingredients:

- 1 cup of honey
- 2 tablespoons of dandelion
- 2 tablespoons of nettle
- 2 tablespoons of yarrow leaves
- 1 teaspoon of thyme

Process:

a. Put the dandelion, nettle, yarrow leaves and thyme in a mortar and use a pestle pound them until they turn into uniform paste.
b. Add the honey and stir well until the mixture blends.
c. Pour the tonic into an airtight jar and store in a warm place for a day before you use it. Take 1-2 teaspoons of the tonic in the morning and in the evening before bed.

26. Eyebrow Oil

To stimulate your eyebrow growth, use this oil.

Ingredients:

- 1 teaspoon of rosemary oil
- 1 teaspoon of pine oil
- 1 teaspoon of olive oil

- 1 teaspoon of lavender oil
- 1 teaspoon of lemon essential oil
- 1 teaspoon of sandalwood essential oil

Process:

a. Mix the oils together and apply the concoction onto your eyebrows daily before bedtime.

27. Hair oil

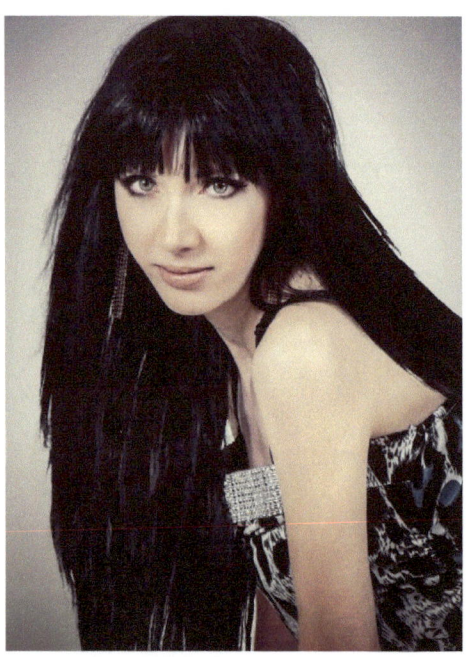

This hair oil helps to stimulate blood circulation and nourishes the hair roots. It promotes thick, strong, smooth and shiny hair.

Ingredients:

- ½ cup of sesame oil
- 2 tablespoon of black pepper
- 2 garlic cloves
- 1 tablespoon of cumin seeds
- 1 small piece of ginger

Process:

a. Slightly crush the garlic and ginger.
b. Heat up the sesame oil in a small pan until it is hot then add the black pepper and cumin seeds.
c. Add the garlic and ginger then let the mixture simmer for a while.
d. Take off the pan from the stove and let the concoction cool.
e. Store the oil in a dark glass bottle.

To use the hair oil, warm it up first until it is moderately warm then massage it onto scalp. Leave it in place for 15-30 minutes then rinse with a detergent-free shampoo. Use the remedy on weekly basis for optimum results.

28. Healthy Smoothie

This smoothie is a remedy for almost all ailments including; reducing bloating, detoxifies, cures indigestion, cures chronic inflammation, enhances energy level, treats acne, increases metabolism, lowers cholesterol, balances body pH and leaves the skin smooth and radiant. For maximum results, drink the smoothie every morning on an empty stomach.

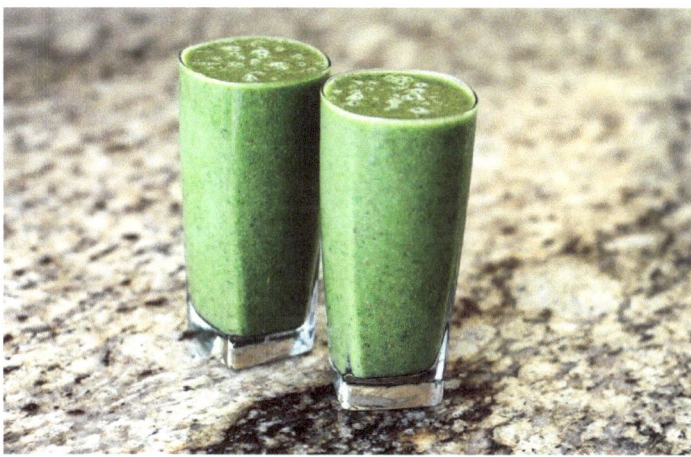

Ingredients:

- 1 tablespoon apple cider vinegar
- 1 small fresh lemon
- 1/8 cayenne pepper
- 1 tablespoon of turmeric powder
- 1 tablespoon of cinnamon powder
- 1 cup of water
- ½ inch stick of ginger

Optional:

- 1 small grapefruit
- 1 tablespoon of raw honey

Process:

a. Use the juicer to extract the juices from the lemon and grapefruit.
b. Put all the ingredients in a cup and pour in boiling water.
c. Let the concoction steep until it is cool enough for your liking.
d. Stir the mixture then drink it up.

29. Oil pulling

Oil pulling or oil gargling is a detoxification technique that uses unrefined vegetable oil such as olive oil, sesame oil, sunflower oil or coconut oil as mouthwash to get rid of toxins from your teeth and mouth. Vegetable oils contain natural antibacterial that fights bacteria and other toxins therefore cleansing your mouth; they flush the toxins before they find their way into the blood stream and cause skin problem such acne. Benefits of oil pulling include preventing bad breath, glowing skin, decrease headache, cure insomnia, heal ulcers, treat toothache, boosts memory, cure bronchitis and other mouth infections such as gum disease and cavities, gives energy, keeping the heart fit and treating chronic fatigue.

Oil pulling method:

1) Put 1 tablespoon of vegetable oil into your mouth.
2) Rinse your mouth by moving the oil around and through your teeth for 15-20 minutes.
3) Do not gurgle the liquid to prevent swallowing it.
4) Spit out the oil and rinse your mouth warm water mixed with table salt. Make sure you rinse thoroughly so as not leave any toxin-infiltrated oil traces in your mouth.

Make sure you perform oil pulling on an empty stomach in the mornings.

30. Lavender, Chamomile and Lemon Bubble Bath Recipe

Ingredients:

- 1 ½ cups of liquid castile soap
- ½ tablespoon of white sugar
- 2 tablespoons of glycerine
- 5 drops lavender essential oil
- 1 drop of chamomile essential oil
- 4 drops of lemon essential oil

Process:

a. Put all the ingredients in a large bowl and stir well until the sugar dissolves.
b. Store the bubble bath in a dark glass bottle and keep in a cool, dark place.
c. Let the bubble bath sit for 24 hours before using it.
d. Pour in ¼ cup of the bubble bath under running water and relax to enjoy the scent as it boosts your mood.

When mixing essential oils, avoid using plastic bowls as it easily absorbs the oils' odour.

Essential Oils

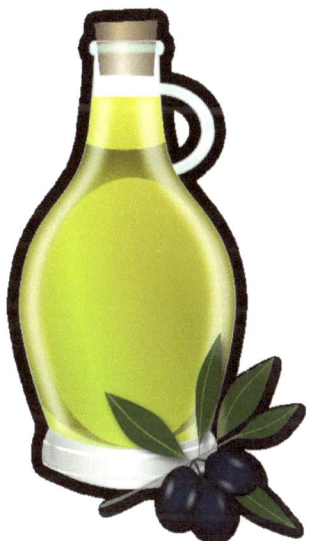

Essential oil also known as volatile oil is a concentrated hydrophobic solution extracted from plants and containing aroma combinations of the plant it is made from. Essential oil contains the essence of the plant and usually extracted using the distillation method. They are popular due to their therapeutic, medicinal and beautifying properties and as such are mostly used to make cosmetics, perfumes, soaps, for body massaging, as food and drink flavourings, to add aroma to incense. Even though our skin produces sebum, natural oil, we need to nourish and moisturise it frequently with natural or pure organic plant oils.

Historically, some medical professionals have sworn about the intrinsic value of essential oils in medical applications and as such some people have continued using them in skin treatments and other health remedies based entirely on historical reports for these tasks. Most countries regulate claims regarding the efficiency and effectiveness of essential oils in treating cancers.

Below are some of the popular essential oils:

Argan oil: It is rich in Vitamin E and also contains fatty acids which are good in treating various skin conditions such premature ageing and it also used to protect the skin, hair and nails against severe conditions and also nourishes the skin.

Bergamot: It is rich in anti-viral and antibacterial properties. It is usually used in acne, blemish and oily skin treatments.

Black Pepper: Its benefits include accelerating digestive system and strengthening the muscles. It also assists in reducing aching muscles, repairing old wounds and weakening muscles, and healing backache.

Carrot seed: It is extracted from the seed of the carrot plant. This oil is beneficial to the skin because it rejuvenates dry, aged, and wrinkled skin. It is rich in antioxidants which assists in reducing the effects of aging and protect the skin from free radicals.

Cedar wood: It assists in alleviating congestion, coughs and skin irritation. It is also good for conditioning scalp.

Chamomile: Its anti-inflammation property helps in soothing skin irritation and it is also good in treating stress.

Eucalyptus: Assists in urinary and respiratory problems. It can be used as cold or hot compress to the body to relieve inflammation in cases like muscular pain and arthritis.

Frankincense: It is used to treat depression and anxiety, muscle stiffness, ulcers, coughs and colds. It is also used as eye makeup (kohl).

Geranium: It is a remedy for premenstrual syndrome (PMS) and menopausal disorder. It also eases skin problems such as acne and skin discoloration.

Grapefruit: It is rich in vitamin C and it is a good airborne antiseptic. It can be used as remedy for congested skin and acne.

Jasmine: Its antiseptic properties help in infections and reduce the change of open wound becoming infected. It is also a remedy for reducing scarring and stretch marks, protecting the skin from free radicals. It moisturises and nourishes all types of skins.

Lavender: It is a great remedy for athlete's foot, wounds, scalds, blisters and other skin conditions such as acne due to its antiviral, antibacterial and antifungal properties.

Lemon grass oil: It is extracted through the method of steam distillation of dried lemongrass. Its benefits include renewing ligaments and the connective tissue, a tissue that supports, connects, or separates various forms of tissues and organs of the body. It is also good in treating cellulite, lessening excessive perspiration and digestive system conditions. It promotes circulation, cures respiratory and sinus ailments, and lowers high cholesterol.

Myrrh: This oil have anti-inflammatory, antioxidant, antiseptic, antiviral and astringent properties and therefore, its uses are numerous; it can be used to treat fungal infections such as athlete's foot, vaginal thrush, eczema and ringworms; to cure tooth and gum diseases, diarrhoea, ulcers, and skin infections such as stretch marks, wrinkles, and to repair cracked skin.

Neroli: This essential oil is also known as orange blossom oil and is extracted from orange blossom flower. Because of its antidepressant properties, this oil is used as a remedy for anxiety and depression. It also have antiseptic, antibacterial, antiviral, antispasmodic and hypertensive properties which assists in alleviating labour pains, PMS, menstrual cramps; fighting bacterial infections, chronic diarrhoea; improving circulation and reduces high blood pressure, and because it stimulates the renewal of skin cells and promotes healing it is therefore used in treating skin conditions such as thread veins, cracked and dry skin, wrinkles and scars marks.

Nutmeg: Due to its anti-inflammatory properties, this essential oil is mostly used for curing arthritis pain, soreness and muscle and joint pains. It also helps in curing indigestion, vomiting and nausea.

Rosehip seed oil: It is extracted from a wild rose known as Rosa Mosqueta. The oil contains vitamin C, omega-3 fatty acid (linoleic acid), omega-6 fatty acid (linoleic acid), omega-9 fatty acid (oleic acid) and antioxidants. It is assists in reducing wrinkles and fine lines, protects the skin from free radical damage produced by UV radiation, and moisturises the dry skin treating scars and acne.

Rosemary: It assists to cure hair loss by stimulating hair growth, cleansing the kidney, easing muscle pain and detoxification.

Sage: It is good in boosting metabolism; alleviating PMS and menstrual cramps, treating skin ailments such as itchy and oily skin, treating dandruff and assists in diminishing scar appearances.

Sandalwood: This oil is extracted from the heartwood of the sandalwood tree. It is used to treat urinary tract infections, cold sores, diarrhoea, and acne; promotes skin cell growth and slows down the appearance of wrinkles and reduces scar marks. It possesses antidepressant properties and it is also a sedative which makes it a good remedy for insomnia and it is used in meditation to help relaxing.

Tea tree oil: This oil is used to alleviate infections such as bronchitis, sinus, ringworms, athlete's foot, tonsillitis, gum diseases, flu and colds and cure skin problems like acne and soreness, reduce swelling or scar tissue and heals wounds due to its antiseptic, antifungal and anti-inflammation properties. It also revitalises the scalp, controls the sebum produced and treats dandruff.

Ylang ylang: It is used to increase both men's and women's libido, combat pre-mature aging conditions by regenerating skin cells, treating skin ailments such as acne and blemish, stimulates hair growth, inhibiting wrinkles and fine lines, and cures insomnia, depression and anxiety.

Avoid storing essential oils in plastic bottles as they can dissolve them.

Carrier Oils

Carrier oil is a vegetable oil or base oil. It mostly used to dilute essential oil before they are applied to the skin in aromatherapy and massage. Carrier oils carry the essential oil onto the skin and they do not evaporate like essential oils. Unlike essential oils, carrier oils do not have concentrated aroma but mostly are odourless or have sweet, mild distinctive smell.

When blending carrier oil with essential oils, always make sure that the carrier oil is natural, unadulterated and not rancid. Keep the oils in dark glass bottles and store in cool, dark place, away from strong light to slow down rancidification. Some oils can be stored in refrigerator to prolong their shelf lives and retard rancidification and may turn cloudy or solidify and prior to use, so they may need to be taken out of refrigerator for some time before they go back to room temperature. There are varieties of carrier oils available but each offers various therapeutic properties and characteristics and choosing oil usually depends on the remedial benefits required such as the area being massaged. There two main processes of producing carrier oils; cold-pressing and maceration. Carrier oils of distinguished quality produced through cold-pressing method are popularly used for culinary consumption as well as in massage use.

Almond Oil (sweet): It is made from dried kernels of almond tree. This versatile is good for nourishing dry skin, reducing skin irritation, inflammation and muscular aches and pains.

Aloe Vera Oil: It is extracted from aloe vera plant. It promotes the body's immune system, assists in easing scarring, eases arthritis pain, speed wound healing and enhances blood circulation. Its anti-inflammatory properties help in infections.

Avocado Oil: It is extracted from avocado seed. This aroma-less oil contains omega-3 fatty acids, high amount of vitamin A and B and is great remedy for dehydrated, sensitive and dry skin. Its anti-inflammatory properties help in treating eczema.

Grape seed Oil: It is usually extracted from the seeds of wine grapes. Its anti-inflammatory properties make it one of the remedy for treating rheumatoid arthritis pain, it promotes circulation, and it contains linoleic acid which is beneficial to diabetic people. This oil assists in easing health conditions such haemorrhoids (also known as piles), varicose and spider veins by repairing and nourishing damaged or broken blood vessels and capillaries.

Hazelnut Oil: It is extracted from hazelnuts and contains vitamin B and E, oleic acid and protein. This astringent oil assists in absorbing excess oil from the skin and the pores, it also has antibacterial properties that help in treating blackheads and pimples.

Olive Oil: It is acquired from the fruits of olive tree and it usually used for cooking, making soap and cosmetic products. It is a source of vitamin A and E which protect the skin from harsh weather conditions and also contains linoleic acid which nourishes and hydrates the skin. It has antibiotic, anti-inflammatory and healing properties which assist in preventing stretch marks (which is why it is a good practise to apply it on the belly during pregnancy) and treating scars grazes. The oil contains antioxidants that nullify the effects of free radicals such as aging signs and skin cancer.

Sesame Seed Oil: This oil is extracted from the seed of sesame plant. Sesame oil is rich in vitamin E which contains antioxidant that can protect the skin from free radicals and oxidation. It is also used to promote blood circulation, restore damaged skin cells, prevents the appearances of wrinkles and fine lines, sooth and moisturise the skin. Its anti-inflammatory helps in preventing bacterial infections and skin conditions such as eczema.

Kukui Oil (Hawaiian): This oil is rich in linoleic and linoleic acids and can be absorbed into the skin with leaving greasy residue. It contains omega-3 fatty acids, it used as a remedy for dehydrated, damaged, mature and dry skin. Its anti-inflammatory properties help in treating eczema, sunburn, scars and acne.

Castor Oil: This oil is normally used in herbal treatment to boosts immunity and for liver detoxification. It is also used for aromatherapy bath oils and put in dry skin and eczema treatment recipes.

Jojoba Oil: It is normally used for hair and scalp treatment. This oil is also used for cosmetics and perfumery and also to extend the shelf life of other blends.

Index

Also by Thato Gaboitsiwe

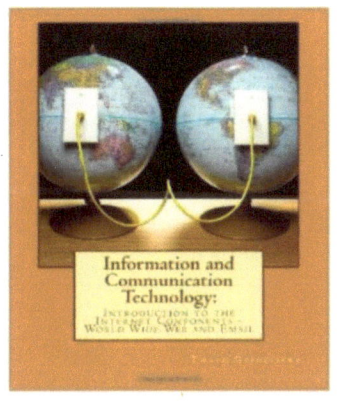

Information and Communication Technology: Introduction to the Internet Components - World Wide Web and Email(Available from Amazon.com)

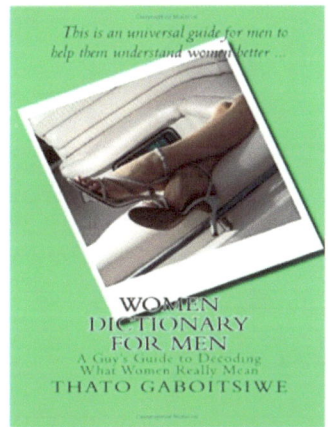

Woman Dictionary For Men:
A Guy's Guide to Decoding What Women Really Mean (Available from Amazon.com)

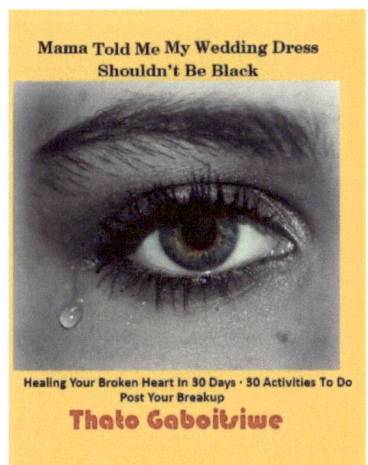

Mama Told me my Wedding Dress Shouldn't be Black: Healing Your Broken Heart in 30 Days • 30 Activities to do Post Your Breakup
(Available from Lulu.com)

My Morning Beauty Regime:

_____

_____

_____

_____

_____

_____

_____

My Evening Beauty Regime:

_____

_____

_____

_____

_____

_____

My Allergies:

_____

_____

_____